Cross

1,000 WOD's To Make You Fitter, Faster, Stronger

TJ Williams

© **Copyright 2015 by HRD Publishing**

All rights Reserved. No part of this book may be reproduced in any form without permission in writing from the author. Reviewers may quote brief passages in reviews.

Table of Contents

Introduction 5
What is Cross Training? 6
Benefits to Cross Training 8
How to use this book 10
Workout Programming 12
    Workout Frequency 12
    2 days on, 1 day off Program 14
    3 days on, 1 day off Program 15
    Workout Configuration 16
Terminology 17
Preparations 20
Beginner WODs 23
    Bodyweight WODs / Little to No Equipment 23
    Basic Barbell WODs 28
    Running WODs 31
    Single Element WODs 40
    Double Element WODs 48
Intermediate WODs 66
    Intermediate Mixed WODs 66
    Gymnastics WODs 77
    Rowing WODs 80
    Swimming WODs 88
    Kettlebell WODs 94
    Dumbbell WODs 100
    Benchmark WODs 105
    EMOM (Every minute on the minute) WODs 110

AMRAP WODs	117
Triple Element WODs	139
Tabata WODs	151
Advanced WODs	**155**
Olympic Lifting WODs	155
Strongman WODs	160
Powerlifting WODs	166
Heros WODs	168
Chipper WODs	198
Create Your Own WODs	**217**
Cool Down	**219**
Summary	**220**
About the Author	**221**
Another Title by TJ Williams	**222**

Introduction

This book is your one-stop guide to Cross Training. This book will not only introduce you to this amazingly effective and often transformative sport, but it offers you 1,000 sample workouts to choose from throughout the text! Anyone can find their place in the world of Cross Training, as the workouts are widely varied, being pulled from aspects of many different sports. If you are coming to this book with a desire to learn more about the sport and get started, use the text as an introduction and continue to refer to the WODs as you become a more seasoned Cross Training athlete. If you are already a Cross Training athlete, you will find numerous workouts to match your fitness level, and likely challenge you to continue to increase your level of performance.

The short duration, high intensity WODs (workouts of the day) are what define the sport of Cross Training. This book breaks down 1,000 WODs into Beginner, Intermediate, and Advanced workout categories. Within each of these categories you will find several more subcategories, encompassing all of the sports that influence Cross Training, and allowing for anyone to find plenty of WODs of interest.

This book will also show you how to design your on WODs. So, once you've worked your way through all 1,000 WODs, you can continue to develop your own. The pain never ends!

This book isn't just about the WODs. I focus on what Cross Training is, workout frequency, implementing a weekly or monthly training plan, and the often overlooked warm ups (Preparations) and cool downs.

No matter your fitness level or athletic interests, you will not be disappointed with what this WOD manual can provide. Take your time getting familiar with what the text has to offer or dive right in. It is really up to. Just remember to be safe, warm-up, cool down, and have fun as you let Cross Training bring you to a level of fitness and performance that you never even knew to be possible!

What is Cross Training?

Cross Training is, simply put, all around exercise combining elements of cardio, strength training and gymnastics, which are then broken down further into hundreds of varieties and combined in new ways. It is an inclusive approach to training that draws from a variety of disciplines to create a dynamic and vigorous workout that is incredibly productive and effective. Its broad approach to method allows for generally improved fitness, attained by participation in comprehensive training sessions that are short, varied, and highly intense.

A Cross Training workout will incorporate elements of strength training, Olympic weightlifting, body building, calisthenics, girevoy sport, boxing, track and field, gymnastics, and other cardiovascular exercise, with the goal of improving general fitness. All of these different elements are mixed up into a cocktail that allow the athlete to find a higher level of overall fitness than can be achieved through exclusively participating in sport-specific training. An athlete is asking more from his or her body when participating in Cross Training than they would with an unvaried approach to fitness. This means that the body's level of fitness essentially has no choice but to improve in a more balanced way. Several goals can be pursued simultaneously in one workout, including, for example, gaining muscle, improving cardiovascular health, losing weight, and improving footwork.

A Cross Training workout can be done in a variety of locations with the amount of equipment that is on hand. Due to the wide variety of options for a Cross Training workout, a workout of the day (WOD) can be completed at a gym, at home, outside, or even in a hotel room. Workouts range from those done with no equipment at all, to those utilizing several pieces of equipment. Like the different components of Cross Training, the equipment used also comes from multiple discipline sources. Pull-up bars, jump ropes, kettle bells, rowing machines, medicine balls, plyo boxes, gymnastics rings, and barbells are all included in the standard equipment utilized in Cross Training.

Cross Training is an approach to exercise that can benefit individuals of all levels of fitness. Whether you are just starting out on your fitness journey or are looking to add something new to your established routine, you will find benefits with the addition of Cross Training to your week. How you want to approach adding Cross Training to your life is up to you, but the following chapters will help to guide you on your way to a healthier, better conditioned you.

Benefits to Cross Training

If you are consistent with your workouts and put in the time and effort, physical and mental benefits that you can see from Cross Training are huge. You will look better, feel better, and have an overall more positive attitude towards your health when you incorporate Cross Training into your fitness routine.

- You will see the positive physical effects of increased conditioning:
    - Improved endurance and stamina
    - Improved strength and speed
    - Improved flexibility and agility
    - Improved balance and coordination
- You will also see positive mental effects:
    - Improved self-esteem and confidence as you see yourself setting and then surpassing your goals.
    - Improved inner strength as you realize how tough you really can be.
    - You will develop a belief that nothing is impossible for you to achieve if you work at it, because after all, with Cross Training you will reach goals you thought were impossible on a regular basis.
    - You will never get bored with your workouts because there is a never-ending variety of options available to you in the world of Cross Training
- There are many other benefits too:
    - Cross Training is an affordable fitness option, as it does not require a lot of equipment to have an effective workout.

- - You will not be stuck paying for a personal trainer or *another* unnecessary gym membership when you have effective workouts available to you through Cross Training.
  - You will not waste hours at the gym when you can get powerful and lasting results in under an hour per workout in your favorite workout spot.
- The established athlete can find a new level of fitness in his or her body, as well as in his or her performance in an established sport:
  - The athlete can become a healthier, more complete competitor due to the broad and inclusive approach taken by Cross Training. For example, a runner that has not traditionally worked strength into his or her routine will find improvements in endurance due to the addition of Cross Training.
  - An already established athlete can also use Cross Training to aid in recovery for over-used muscles that can often occur in specialized training. Other muscles are strengthened, as those that are overworked are allowed the opportunity to heal, which can then aid in improving overall performance for the athlete.

No matter where you are in your fitness journey, Cross Training has virtually endless benefits to offer. It will bring you to an improved level of fitness no matter where you start. And eventually, you may find yourself reaching goals that you did not even know you would ever have.

How to use this book

This book is meant to be your ultimate guide to Cross Training. If you are interested in learning more about this unique approach to fitness and seeing all that it has to offer, you can read it cover-to-cover. You may also just want to read the introductory sections and then use the WOD sections as a reference. It is flexible and able to be tailored to your needs, just as Cross Training is flexible and meant to be tailored to your goals.

There are, however, some important guidelines that you will need to follow no matter your fitness level or goals:

1. *Always* warm-up. Either use one of the suggested Preparations, or do your own warm-up. It is important that you get your body ready to work before jumping into these workouts. They are short in duration, but they are high intensity and you must allow your body the chance to warm-up to avoid injury. The general rule of thumb for a basic warm up is 5-10 mins with an elevated heart rate (not out of breath).

2. Follow-up your warm-up with light mobility work or stretching to start. Mimic some of the movements that you're going to be doing during the WOD. If you WOD involves Squats and press ups, warm up with squats and press ups. Ideally, do a less intense version of the movement ie. Half squats, or press ups on a Box/Wall. Also incorporate static holds in the bottom positions for 5-10 seconds.

3. Select your specific workout from one of the WOD sections provided.

4. Keep a record of your workout to track your progress. *This will be especially important as you continue with Cross Training in the future so that you can see your improvements. Depending on the WOD, you'll need to record one or more of the following:*

    - Record Times
    - Record Reps

- Record Rounds
- Record Weight(s)
- Date of the Workout

End with a cool down, and do not forget to hydrate. And congratulations on completing your workout! Keep up the good work!

Workout Programming

This book contains 1,000 WOD's, which offers great variety for you, but where do you start?

This chapter will explore the common programming options you can utilize, how you can implement an even split of body weight training, barbell work and CV into your routine for total body fitness, and how you can select particular workouts to meet your needs.

Workout Frequency

Your workout frequency (how many times you do a Cross Training workout during the week) will vary depending on your goals and your participation in other forms of athletics. However, here are some general guidelines to help you select the right one for you:

- For complete beginners, start Cross Training 3 days per week with at least a day off in between WODs. For example, a general Mon, Wed, Fri - WODs with the weekend off is a great place to start out.

- Over the next 3 to 6 months, work up to 4 or 5 days a week. A lot of beginners rush this phase and I would urge caution here. Take your time. Rest days are hugely important, especially when you're just starting out. You need to rest to allow your body to recover, grow and prepare for the next workout.

- You can work up to a 2 day on, 1 day off frequency, and eventually, a 3 day on, and 1 day off maximum. For example, Mon, Tue - workouts, Wed - rest day. Thu, Fri - workouts, Sat - rest day and so on. I wouldn't recommend working out more than this, and it may take you 6 to 12 months to work up to this. Listen to your body!

- Rest an extra day if you are feeling very sore. The frequencies above are general guides. You must eventually learn how to listen to your body and respond accordingly. There's a difference between feeling tired, and being completely rundown. Training when you're tired is fine. Training when your body is rundown is asking for illness or injury. You'll generally find an extra rest day or a workout replacement by a gentle walk will do wonders to your recovery, and allow you to hit the next WOD with more energy. Leave your ego at the door and listen to your body!

- Use variety in your training. Don't do the same couple of WODs every time you workout, and make sure to use WODs that hit different muscle groups. For example, don't do a lower body workout three days in a row. If you're following a Mon, Wed, Fri split - Train your legs Mon and Fri, and your upper body on Wed to rest your legs. With the 3 day on and 1 day off approach. You can use a push, pull, and leg split - Predominantly 'pushing WODs' include Press ups, and Handstand Push ups, 'pulling WODs' include a lot of pull ups and rowing, and 'leg WODs' might include more running or squats.

- Make sure to have a balance of strength, gymnastics and cardio throughout the week. Try to incorporate this into your weekly routine.

Cross Training is all about variety. When you're reviewing how to set up a training plan for yourself, consider variance and randomness. Your ideal training plan should become something that is **not** routine in structure. You want a healthy mix of Barbell work, body weight exercises and CV conditioning during each week to progress in all areas. This will also ensure you're improving your weaknesses. We all have weaknesses, and we are naturally inclined to avoid them. Cross Training is geared to attacking your weaknesses with the same vigor as your strengths. This will enable you to become a more well-rounded athlete.

To demonstrate what a nice well-rounded training plan might look like, let me show you a 2 day on, 1 day off schedule.

Key

BB = Barbell, Dumbbell, Kettlebell work (Squats, Presses, Cleans, Kettlebell Swings, Dumbbell Press etc.)

BW = Bodyweight exercises (Press ups, Pull ups, Sit ups, Handstand Press, Dips, Air Squat etc.)

CV = Cardio Vascular exercise (Running, Rowing, Swimming, Skipping etc.)

2 days on, 1 day off Program

Day 1 – BB, CV

Day 2 – BW

Day 3 – Rest Day

Day 4 – CV, BW

Day 5 – BB

Day 6 – Rest Day

Day 7 – BB, BW

Day 8 – CV

Day 9 – Rest Day

The program above has an equal split of covering each form of exercise 3 times in 9 days. Each format has a single day priority and 2 shared days. You just repeat the process every 9 days.

You can use the same process for 3 days on and 1 day off. You just need to adjust the daily formats to a single, double and triple instead. I've demonstrated what this would look like below:

3 days on, 1 day off Program

Day 1 – BB

Day 2 – BW, CV

Day 3 – BB, BW, CV

Day 4 – Rest Day

Day 5 – BW

Day 6 – CV, BB

Day 7 – BW, CV, BB

Day 8 – Rest Day

Day 9 – CV

Day 10 – BW, BB

Day 11 – CV, BW, BB

Day 12 – Rest Day

The program above has an equal split of covering each form of exercise 6 times in 12 days. As you can tell this isn't for the faint-hearted! For 3 extra days, you do twice the amount of work as the 2 day on, 1 day off program. Each format has a single, double and triple day priority. You repeat the process every 12 days.

You are not restricted to these schedules. Find a schedule that you can commit to on a consistent basis, and map out the formats like I have above to allow you to focus time on all exercise formats.

Workout Configuration

Once you have your schedule in place you can go into more detail on the actual WOD itself.

On a single BB day you can focus on low rep, heavy weight exercises for strength, like finding your 3 rep max for the Back Squat.

On a single BW day you can work on the technical aspects of Muscle ups, Pull ups, Push ups, Sit ups etc. Or perform a bodyweight only WOD.

On a single CV day you'll perform a prolonged, steady distance effort on the rowing machine, in the pool or during a run.

When you're on double and triple format days you can incorporate some of the many WOD's I've provided for you in this book. I would once again encourage you to use variety in your selection. Balance your program with task and time orientated WOD's.

Task WODs – The reps and exercises are set and you're against the clock. (eg. 5 rounds for time: 1 round = 5x Burpees and 20x kettlebell swings)

Timed WODs – The tasks are fixed, but there are unlimited rounds until the time runs out. (eg. As Many Rounds As Possible in 20 mins: 5x ½ body weight cleans, 10x push ups and 400m run)

Train your weaknesses, and as a general rule of thumb, if you don't enjoy an exercise or WOD, do more of it! Make your weaknesses strong. The ultimate Cross Trainers are individuals with a broad base of skill and ability in all areas.

Terminology

These are some common acronyms that you will need to know in Cross Training:

General

- AMRAP = As Many Reps/Rounds as Possible
- WOD = Workout of the Day
- WO = Workout
- KB = Kettlebell
- PR = Personal Record
- Rep = Repetitions (of an exercise)
- Set = Number of Repetitions
- Rx'd = WOD done as prescribed (written) with no adjustments
- RM = Rep Max/Repetition Maximum/Most weight you can lift for a certain number of repetitions. (*i.e. 10 RM is the most you can left 10 times*)
- Subbed = Substituted (when you use one exercise in the place of a prescribed one that you cannot do in a certain workout)
- ATG = Ass to Grass
- EMOM = Every minute on the Minute

Exercises

- AHAP = As heavy as possible
- BB = Barbell

- BP = Bench Press
- BS = Back Squat
- BW (BWT) = Body Weight
- C2B = Chest to Bar
- CLN = Clean
- C&J = Clean and Jerk
- DL = Deadlift
- DU = Double unders
- FS = Front Squat
- GHD = Glute Ham Developer
- H2H = Hand to Hand
- HSPU = Hand Stand Push-up
- HSQ = Hang Squat (Snatch or Clean)
- KTE = Knees to Elbows
- MP = Military Press
- MU = Muscle Ups
- OHS = Overhead Squat
- PC = Power Clean
- PP = Push Press
- POOD = Russian measurement for kettlebells (1 pood = 36 lbs)
- PSN = Power Snatch
- PU = Pull-up

- SLDL = Straight leg dead lift
- SDHP = Sumo deadlift high pull
- SN = Snatch
- SU = Single Unders
- SQ = Squat
- TGU = Turkish get-up
- TTB = Toes to Bar

Preparations

Preparations, or Warm-ups, are very important before you begin your full Cross Training workout. Cross Training is fast and intense and you want your body ready to work hard so that you:

1. Perform at your best
2. Prevent injury

A warm-up is meant to get your blood flowing to the relevant muscles for your workout, including your heart. You also want to get the relevant joints moving and warm. It is best to start at about a 25% effort until you start sweating, proceed with some mobility work, and then begin your workout.

I have provided some examples of Preparations/Warm-ups that can be used before you begin your day's WOD. Some require ore equipment than others. However, you may also choose to do your own favorite Warm-up. A good rule of thumb if you are designing your own Preparation is to complete 2 – 3 sets of 10 – 15 reps for 3 – 4 exercises. The complexity of the Warm-up is not what matters. The most important thing is to make sure that all of the relevant muscles are prepared to do the work that is asked of them. Once that is complete, then stretch and complete some mobility work. In total, between your warm-up and your mobility work, you should spend about 15 minutes on your preparation for a Cross Training workout.

Example Preparation #1
400m run
10 squats
3x 10m bear Crawls
3x 10m lunges

Example Preparation #2
25x each with a PVC/broomstick:
Shoulder dislocates
Shoulder press

Overhead squat
Romanian deadlift
Bent row
Good mornings

Example Preparation #3
400m run
10 squats
400m run
10 press ups

Example Preparation #4
1 round
Jog 5 minutes
Row 3 minutes
Jump rope 2 minutes
Walk 1 minute

Example Preparation #5
Run 4x50m; down forward, back reverse
Then, 2 rounds of
25m Walking lunge, forward
25m Walking lunge, backward
15x Push-ups
15x PVC shoulder dislocate

Example Preparation #6
Warm-up: 3 rounds
10x Walking lunges
10x Squats
10x Push-ups
10x Box jumps
Run 100m

Example Preparation #7
Run 4x50m; down forward, back reverse
Then, 2 rounds of
25m Walking lunge, forward
25m Walking lunge, backward
15x Push-ups
15x PVC shoulder dislocate

Example Preparation #8
10x10m shuttle
Then, 2 rounds of
5x/leg Box step-ups (20")
10x Ball slam (20#)
10x Hand-release push-ups

Additional Preparation Ideas
10-15 minutes bicycle
10-15 minutes run
10-15 minutes row
10-15 minutes jump rope

Beginner WODs

Beginner WODs are where you will want to start on your Cross Training journey. These workouts are the easiest to perform. They are ones that do not require as much technical expertise or equipment. They also generally call for fewer reps ad less weight than other WODs. They are best for those starting out, but can also be a valuable tool for a seasoned Cross Training athlete who may be looking for a faster workout, a simpler workout, a lighter day, or a workout not requiring equipment (maybe they are traveling or working out at home). Even though these are considered "beginner" workouts, they are still challenging, so remember to always start your workout with a preparation and mobility work to prevent injury.

Bodyweight WODs / Little to No Equipment

Bodyweight WOD #1
8 rounds, Record time
20 seconds on/10 seconds off
Air squats
Push-ups
Sit-ups
Optional 4th Movement
Burpees

Bodyweight WOD #2 – Breezy
3 rounds
21-15-9x reps
Pull-ups
Push-ups
Sit-ups
Squats

Bodyweight WOD #3
1 round
60x Push-ups
50x Body rows
40x Sit-ups
30x Squats
20x Dips
10x Box jumps
5x Burpees

Bodyweight WOD #4
5 rounds
22x Burpees
22x Pull-ups
22x Sit-ups

Bodyweight WOD #5
Max rounds in 20 minutes
15x Pull-ups
10x Pistols
5x Handstand push-ups (can scale these to a HS kick-ups, push press or KB press)

Bodyweight WOD #6
3 rounds, 50-35-20x reps
Push-ups
Pull-ups
Backward walking lunge steps

Bodyweight WOD #7
3 rounds
Run 400m
25m Burpee broad jumps
25m Walking lunges

25m Burpee broad jumps
25m Bear crawl

Bodyweight WOD #8
1 round
50x Push-ups
10x Star jumps
50x Sit-ups
10x Star jumps
50x Squats
10x Star jumps
50x Body rows
10x Star jumps

Bodyweight WOD #9
10 rounds
10x Walking lunge steps, forward
10x Walking lunge steps, backward
10x Push-ups

Bodyweight WOD #10
5 rounds
20m Handstand walk to a wall
50x Shoulder taps

Bodyweight WOD #11 – Ivan
4 rounds
50x Double-unders
50-40-30-20x Walking lunges
50-40-30-20x Push-ups
50-40-30-20x Sit-ups

Bodyweight WOD #12 – Jimmy
3 rounds

Walking lunge steps 100 ft
10x Handstand push-ups

Bodyweight WOD #13 – Coach Walter
3 rounds
Run 400m
40x Walking lunge steps
30x Sit ups
20x Push ups
10x Burpees

Bodyweight WOD #14
4 rounds
50x Squats
40x Back extensions
30x Push-ups

Bodyweight WOD #15
For time
90x Double unders
50x Walking lunges
40x Push-ups
30x Sit-ups
20x Burpees
10x Handstand push-ups

Bodyweight WOD #16
7 rounds
7x Burpees
7x Sit-ups

Bodyweight WOD #17
1 round
15x Spiderman push-ups

10x Squats
15x Mountain climbers
10x Squats
15x Spartan push-ups
10x Squats
15x Hindu push-ups
10x Squats
15x Dips

Bodyweight WOD #18 – The Runway
For time
400m Burpee broad jumps
400m Walking lunges
Run 400m
400m Bear crawl

Bodyweight WOD #19
For time
3-minute Handstand hold
100x Squats
50m Handstand walk
100x Squats
30x Handstand push-ups

Bodyweight WOD #20
10 rounds
10x Vertical jumps
10x Push-ups

Bodyweight WOD #21
6 RFT
30x Jumping jacks
30x Burpees
100m Walking lunges

Bodyweight WOD #22
20x Inverted burpees
50x Jumping jacks
30x Push-ups

Bodyweight WOD #23
4 RFT
30x Tuck jumps
15x Burpees
10x HSPU

Bodyweight WOD #24
Max rounds in 16 minutes
100m Crab walk
30x Burpees
20x Pull-ups

Bodyweight WOD #25
6 RFT
200m Run
30x Star jumps
200m Run
30x Burpees
20x Sit-ups

Basic Barbell WODs

Basic Barbell WOD #1
15 min to work to 1RM
Back Squat

Basic Barbell WOD #2

10 min to work to 3RM
Back Squat

Basic Barbell WOD #3
10 min to work to 10RM
Back Squat

Basic Barbell WOD #4
12 min to work to 10RM
Back Squat

Basic Barbell WOD #5
12 min to work to 3x3 @ 80%

Basic Barbell WOD #6
12 min to work to 1RM
Front Squat

Basic Barbell WOD #7
12 min to work to 3RM
Front Squat

Basic Barbell WOD #7
12 min to work to 10RM
Front Squat

Basic Barbell WOD #8
12 min to work to 4x4 @ 75%
Front Squat

Basic Barbell WOD #9
10 min to work to heavy but perfect
Overhead Squat

Basic Barbell WOD #10
12 min to work to 3RM
Overhead Squat

Basic Barbell WOD #11
12 min to work to 1RM
Strict press

Basic Barbell WOD #12
12 min to work to 3RM
Strict press

Basic Barbell WOD #12
10 min to work to 1RM
Push Press

Basic Barbell WOD #13
10 min to work to 3RM
Push Press

Basic Barbell WOD #14
15 minutes to work to 1RM
Deadlift

Basic Barbell WOD #15
15 minutes to work to a 3R
Deadlift

Basic Barbell WOD #16
For time
15x SDHP

Basic Barbell WOD #17
15 minutes to work to 1RM

Bench Press

Basic Barbell WOD #18
15 minutes to work to 3RM
Bench Press

Basic Barbell WOD #19
Max Rounds in 20 minutes
Each round 10x Bench Press

Running WODs

Running WOD #1
For time
Run 1 mile
Stop every minute and do 30x jumping jacks

Running WOD #2
For time
Run 1 mile
30x Chest to bar pull-ups

Running WOD #3
3 rounds
Run 200m
25x Push-ups

Running WOD #4
1 round
30x Pull-ups, kipping
Run 400m
12x Pull-ups, strict
Run 400m

5x Pull-ups, weighted (40#/25#)
Run 400m

Running WOD #5
For time
100x Double-unders
Run 1 mile
100x Burpees
Run 1 mile
100x Double-unders

Running WOD #6
10 rounds
20m Walking handstand
Sprint 100m between each set
For time
Run 1 mile
Do 100x squats at 1/2 mile mark

Running WOD #7 – Jared
4 rounds
Run 800m
40x Pull-ups
70x Push-ups

Running WOD #8 - Prison Break
20-19-18-...-3-2-1x
Burpees
Sprint 50m

Running WOD #9 - No Excuses
For time
Run 2km
100s Push-ups

100x Sit-ups
50x Burpees

Running WOD #10 – Capoot
4 rounds
100-75-50-25x Push-ups
Run 800-1200-1600-2000m

Running WOD #11
For time
30x Push-ups
Run 300m
30x Squats
Run 200m
30x Burpees
Run 100m
30x Sit-ups
Run 50m
30x Jumping jacks

Running WOD #12
3 rounds
Run 400m
Muscle-ups 18-15-12x

Running WOD #13
For time
Run 1200-800-400-200-100m
50-40-30-20-10x Push-ups
50-40-30-20-10x Sit-ups

Running WOD #14
For time
Run 1 mile

100x "Bodyblasters" (burpee + pull-up + knees to elbows)
Run 1 mile

Running WOD #15 - The heat
3 rounds
21-15-9x reps, start and finish WOD with 800m run
Handstand push-ups
Burpees
Knees to elbows

Running WOD #16 - Five for the road
10 rounds, start and finish WOD with 1 mile run
20-18-16-14-12-10-8-6-4-2x reps
Pull-ups
Burpees
Push-ups
Sit-ups
Squats

Running WOD #17
For time
Run 1600m
100x Push-ups
Run 800m
75x Squats
Run 400m
50x Sit-ups
Run 200m

Running WOD #18
For time
Run 1/2 mile
50x Push-ups
50x Sit-ups

50x Squats
50x Pull-ups
50x Double-unders
Run 1/2 mile

Running WOD #19 – Little Evil
3 rounds
Run 800m
30x Pull-ups
30x Burpees

Running WOD #20
1 round
Run 1200m
100x Push-ups
150x Sit-ups
200x Squats
Run 1200m

Running WOD #21
For time
Run 1 mile
100x "Bodyblasters" (burpee + pull-up + knees to elbows)
Run 1 mile

Running WOD #22 - Mark Owns
4 rounds
Run 800m
30x Sit-ups
10x Pull-ups

Running WOD #23
3 RFT
Run 800

50x Air squats

Running WOD #24
5 RFT
Run 200m
10x Air squats
10x Push-ups

Running WOD #25
3 RFT
Run 200m
25x Push-ups

Running WOD #26
3 RFT
10x HSPU
Run 200m

Running WOD #27
10-9-8-7-6-5-4-3-2-1 Set of sit-ups
100m sprint between each set

Running WOD #28
10 RFT
10x Push-ups
Run 100m

Running WOD #29
For time
Run 1 mile, lunging 30 steps every minute

Running WOD #30
5 RFT
Run 400m

5 Burpees

Running WOD #31
10 RFT
100m Sprints
10x Sit-ups

Running WOD #32
5 RFT
Run 1 minute
Squat 1 minute

Running WOD #33
3 RFT
Run 400m
50 Air squats
25 Push-ups

Running WOD #34
10 RFT
5x Push-ups with 30 second plebs plank at top
100m dash

Running WOD #35
25x tries at free handstand
Run 1 mile @ 80%

Running WOD #36
For time
50x Walking lunges
800m Run
50 Walking lunges

Running WOD #37

For time
60x Push-ups
400m Run
40x Push-ups
800m Run
20x Push-ups
1 mile Run

Running WOD #38
100x Air squats
75x Sit-ups
50x Box jumps
25x KTEs
400m Run

Running WOD #39 – Michael
3 RFT
800m Run
50x Back extensions
50x Sit-ups

Running WOD #40
5 RFT
200m Run
10x Thrusters

Running WOD #41
18 TTB
200m Run
15x KB Swing

Running WOD #42
4 RFT
25x Power snatches

400m Run

Running WOD #43
5 RFT
400m Run
25x Dips

Running WOD #44
3 RFT
25x Box jumps
15x Wall balls
800m Run

Running WOD #45
3 RFT
1 mile Run
5 Clean and jerks

Running WOD #46
For time
5x OH Presses
25 DUs
5x OH Presses
400m Run
5x OH Presses
400m Run

Running WOD #47
5 RFT
25x Ab mat sit-ups
25x Ring rows
200m Sprint

Running WOD #48

For time
800m Run
25 Air squats
800m Run
1 minute plank

Running WOD #49
3 RFT
600m run
35 KB Swing
15 Jumping pull-ups

Running WOD #50
3 RFT
6 HSPU
400m Run

Single Element WODs

Single Element WOD #1
For time
1600m on a track, using either Bear Crawl, Crab Walk, or Broad Jump to move

Single Element WOD #2
Max reps in 12 minutes
Handstand Push-up

Single Element WOD #3
For time
100x Squats

Single Element WOD #4 - Burpee Heaven

For time
1000x Burpees

This is an incredibly advanced workout that you should take your time working up to. However, it is included here because it requires no equipment and consist of just the one exercise.

Single Element WOD #6 - Death by box

5 rounds
Total reps=score
45 seconds Box jumps (18 inch)
15 seconds rest
45 seconds Box jumps (24 inch)
15 seconds rest
45 seconds Box jumps (30+ inch)
15 seconds rest

Single Element WOD #7 - G.I. Jane

For time
100x Burpee pull-ups

Single Element WOD #8

For time
100m Walking handstand

Single Element WOD #9

Max reps in 12 minutes
Pull-ups, strict

Single Element WOD #10

For time
50x Double Unders

Single Element WOD #11

For time

75x Press ups for time

Single Element WOD #12
For time
100x Wall Balls

Single Element WOD #13
For time
75x Power snatches

Single Element WOD #14
Max reps in 12 minutes
Snatches

Single Element WOD #15
For time
100x Pull-ups

Single Element WOD #16
Max reps in 8 minutes
Pull-ups (weighted for Rx+)

Single Element WOD #17
Max Reps in 8 minutes
Double-unders

Single Element WOD #18
For time
50x Dips

Single Element WOD #19
Max reps in 8 minutes
Dips

Single Element WOD #20
Max reps in 12 minutes
Wall Balls

Single Element WOD #21
Max reps in 12 minutes
Walking lunges with wall ball

Single Element WOD #22
For time
50 Walking lunges with KB (50/35)

Single Element WOD #23
For time
100 Walking lunges (no weight)

Single Element WOD #24
For time
5x Muscle-ups
Rest 3 minutes
5x Muscle-ups
Rest 3 minutes
5x Muscle-ups

Single Element WOD #25
For time
50x Ring rows

Single Element WOD #26
Max reps in 12 minutes
Ring rows

Single Element WOD #27
For time

75x Jumping squats

Single Element WOD #28
Max reps in 12 minutes
Bar facing burpees

Single Element WOD #29
For time
50x Back extensions

Single Element WOD #30
Max reps in 12 minutes
Weighted back extensions

Single Element WOD #31
For time
100x Toes to bar (TTB)

Single Element WOD #32
For time
100x Knees to elbows (KTE)

Single Element WOD #33
For time
75x Push Jerks

Single Element WOD #34
For time
75x Split jerks

Single Element WOD #35
For time
75x Cleans

Single Element WOD #36
For time
50x Clean and Jerk

Single Element WOD #37
Max Reps 12 minutes
OH Walking Lunges (45/25)

Single Element WOD #38
For time
50 Jumping pull-ups

Single Element WOD #39
For time
100 Box jump-overs

Single Element WOD #40
Max reps in 8 minutes
Deadlift (225/155)

Single Element WOD #41
For time
100 Ab mat-sit-ups

Single Element WOD #42
Max reps in 12 minutes
Medicine ball sit-ups

Single Element WOD #43
Max reps in 12 minutes
Push-ups

Single Element WOD #44
Max reps in 12 minutes

Wide arm push-ups

Single Element WOD #45
Max reps in 12 minutes
Triceps push-ups

Single Element WOD #46
For time
50x OH Squats

Single Element WOD #47
Max reps in 12 minutes
KB OH Presses (left then right)

Single Element WOD #48
Max reps in 8 minutes
Thrusters (135/80)

Single Element WOD #49
For time
75x Back squats

Single Element WOD #50
For time
75x Back squats

Single Element WOD #51
Max reps in 12 minutes
Push Press

Single Element WOD #52
Max reps in 8 minutes
OH Press/Strict press

Single Element WOD #53
For time
100 KB Swings

Single Element WOD #54
For time
15x Rope Climb

Single Element WOD #55
For time
250x Press-ups

Single Element WOD #56
For time
50x Burpee thrusters

Single Element WOD #57
For time
100x Pull-up bar kipping

Single Element WOD #58
Max reps in 12 minutes
Hang squat snatches

Single Element WOD #59
Max reps 8 minutes
Butterfly pull-ups

Single Element WOD #60
For time'
100x Goblet squats

Single Element WOD #61
For time

50x Inverted burpees

Single Element WOD #62
Hold plank for 1 minutes
Rest 1 minute
Hold plank for 2 minutes
Rest 1 minute
Hold plank for 3
As you become stronger, increase plank times in 1 minute intervals

Double Element WODs

Double Element WOD #1
5 rounds
25-20-15-10-5x
Hand release push-ups
Box jumps (24/20 inch)

Double Element WOD #2
10 rounds
10-9-8-…-3-2-1x Strict pull-ups
30-27-24-…9-6-3x Push-ups

Double Element WOD #3
10 rounds
Start and finish couplet with 800m run
10x Handstand push-up
10x Pistols

Double Element WOD #4 - Cottage cheese and flying squirrels
3 rounds

50x Ring dips
100x Squats
Sweet pea

Double Element WOD #5
1 round
50x Double unders
10x Box jumps
40x Double unders
20x Box jumps
30x Double unders
30x Box jumps
20x Double unders
40x Box jumps
10x Double unders
50x Box jumps

Double Element WOD #6
5 rounds
20x Double unders
15 ft Rope climb, 1 ascent

Double Element WOD #7
Max rounds in 12 minutes
7x Handstand push-ups
12x L pull-ups

Double Element WOD #8
Max rounds in 12 minutes
15 ft Rope climb, 1 ascent
15x Push-ups

Double Element WOD #9
5 rounds

20x Double unders
15 ft Rope climb, 1 ascent

Double Element WOD #10
For time
50x Double unders
10x Handstand push-ups
40x Double unders
8x Handstand push-ups
30x Double unders
6x Handstand push-ups
20x Double unders
4x Handstand push-ups
10x Double unders
2x Handstand push-ups

Double Element WOD #11
8 rounds
30-sec Handstand
10x Squats

Double Element WOD #12
Escalating/Deescalating WOD
Record time
50 push ups
20 air squats
40 push ups
40 air squats
30 push ups
60 air squats
20 push ups
80 air squats
10 push ups
100 air squats

Double Element WOD #13
21 - 15 - 9
Box Jumps
Sit-ups

Double Element WOD #14
21 - 15 - 9
Box Jumps
Deadlift

Double Element WOD #15
21 - 15 – 9
Box Jumps
TTB

Double Element WOD #16
21 - 15 – 9
Box Jumps
KTE

Double Element WOD #17
21 - 15 - 9
Box Jumps
Walking Lunges

Double Element WOD #18
21 - 15 - 9
Box Jumps
Thrusters

Double Element WOD #19
21 - 15 - 9
Box Jumps

Push Press

Double Element WOD #20
21 - 15 - 9
Box Jumps
OH Press

Double Element WOD #21
21 - 15 - 9
Box Jumps
OH Squat

Double Element WOD #22
21 - 15 - 9
Box Jumps
Back Extensions

Double Element WOD #23
21 - 15 - 9
Box Jumps
Push-ups

Double Element WOD #24
21 - 15 - 9
Box Jumps
Ring rows

Double Element WOD #25
21 - 15 - 9
Box Jumps
Pull-ups

Double Element WOD #26
21 - 15 - 9
Box Jumps

Dips

Double Element WOD #27
21 - 15 - 9
Box Jumps
Wall balls

Double Element WOD #28
21 - 15 - 9
Sit-ups
Double-unders

Double Element WOD #29
21 - 15 - 9
Sit-ups
Single-unders

Double Element WOD #30
21 - 15 - 9
Sit-ups
Deadlift

Double Element WOD #31
21 - 15 - 9
Sit-ups
TTB

Double Element WOD #32
21 - 15 - 9
Sit-ups
KTE

Double Element WOD #33
21 - 15 - 9

Sit-ups
Walking lunges

Double Element WOD #34
21 - 15 - 9
Sit-ups
Thrusters

Double Element WOD #35
21 - 15 - 9
Sit-ups
Push press

Double Element WOD #36
21 - 15 - 9
Sit-ups
OH press

Double Element WOD #37
21 - 15 - 9
Sit-ups
OH squat

Double Element WOD #38
21 - 15 - 9
Sit-ups
Push-ups

Double Element WOD #39
21 - 15 - 9
Sit-ups
Pull-ups

Double Element WOD #40

21 - 15 - 9
Sit-ups
Dips

Double Element WOD #41
21 - 15 - 9
Sit-ups
Wall balls

Double Element WOD #42
21 - 15 - 9
Sit-ups
Ring rows

Double Element WOD #43
21 - 15 - 9
Double-unders
Deadlift

Double Element WOD #44
21 - 15 - 9
Double-unders
TTB

Double Element WOD #45
21 - 15 - 9
Double-unders
KTE

Double Element WOD #46
21 - 15 - 9
Double-unders
Walking lunges

Double Element WOD #47
21 - 15 - 9
Double-unders
Thrusters

Double Element WOD #48
21 - 15 - 9
Double-unders
Push press

Double Element WOD #49
21 - 15 - 9
Double-unders
Push press

Double Element WOD #50
21 - 15 - 9
Double-unders
OH press

Double Element WOD #51
21 - 15 - 9
Double-unders
OH Squat

Double Element WOD #52
21 - 15 - 9
Double-unders
Back extensions

Double Element WOD #53
21 - 15 - 9
Double-unders
Push-ups

Double Element WOD #54
21 - 15 - 9
Double-unders
Pull-ups

Double Element WOD #55
21 - 15 - 9
Double-unders
Wall balls

Double Element WOD #56
21 - 15 - 9
Double-unders
Ring rows

Double Element WOD #57
21 - 15 - 9
Single-unders
Deadlift

Double Element WOD #58
21 - 15 - 9
Single-unders
TTB

Double Element WOD #59
21 - 15 - 9
Single-unders
KTE

Double Element WOD #60
21 - 15 - 9
Single-unders

Walking lunges

Double Element WOD #61
21 - 15 - 9
Single-unders
Thrusters

Double Element WOD #62
21 - 15 - 9
Single-unders
Push press

Double Element WOD #63
21 - 15 - 9
Single-unders
Push press

Double Element WOD #64
21 - 15 - 9
Single-unders
OH press

Double Element WOD #65
21 - 15 - 9
Single-unders
OH Squat

Double Element WOD #66
21 - 15 - 9
Single-unders
Back extensions

Double Element WOD #67
21 - 15 - 9

Single-unders
Push-ups

Double Element WOD #68
21 - 15 - 9
Single-unders
Pull-ups

Double Element WOD #69
21 - 15 - 9
Single-unders
Wall balls

Double Element WOD #70
21 - 15 - 9
Single-unders
Ring rows

Double Element WOD #71
21 - 15 - 9
TTB
Deadlift

Double Element WOD #72
21 - 15 - 9
TTB
Walking lunges

Double Element WOD #73
21 - 15 - 9
TTB
Push press

Double Element WOD #74

21 - 15 - 9
TTB
OH press

Double Element WOD #75
21 - 15 - 9
TTB
OH squat

Double Element WOD #76
21 - 15 - 9
TTB
Back extensions

Double Element WOD #77
21 - 15 - 9
TTB
Push-ups

Double Element WOD #78
21 - 15 - 9
TTB
Pull-ups

Double Element WOD #79
21 - 15 - 9
TTB
Dips

Double Element WOD #80
21 - 15 - 9
TTB
Dips

Double Element WOD #81
21 - 15 - 9
KTE
Deadlift

Double Element WOD #82
21 - 15 - 9
KTE
Walking lunges

Double Element WOD #83
21 - 15 - 9
KTE
Push press

Double Element WOD #84
21 - 15 - 9
KTE
OH press

Double Element WOD #85
21 - 15 - 9
KTE
OH squat

Double Element WOD #86
21 - 15 - 9
KTE
Back extensions

Double Element WOD #87
21 - 15 - 9
KTE
Push-ups

Double Element WOD #88
21 - 15 - 9
KTE
Pull-ups

Double Element WOD #89
21 - 15 - 9
KTE
Dips

Double Element WOD #90
21 - 15 - 9
KTE
Wall balls

Double Element WOD #91
21 - 15 - 9
Walking lunges
Push press

Double Element WOD #92
21 - 15 - 9
Walking lunges
OH press

Double Element WOD #93
21 - 15 - 9
Walking lunges
OH squat

Double Element WOD #94
21 - 15 - 9
Walking lunges

Back extensions

Double Element WOD #95
21 - 15 - 9
Walking lunges
Push-ups

Double Element WOD #96
21 - 15 - 9
Walking lunges
Pull-ups

Double Element WOD #97
21 - 15 - 9
Walking lunges
Dips

Double Element WOD #98
21 - 15 - 9
Walking lunges
Wall balls

Double Element WOD #99
21 - 15 - 9
Walking lunges
Thrusters

Double Element WOD #100
21 - 15 - 9
Walking lunges
Deadlift

Double Element WOD #101
21 - 15 - 9

Wall balls
Push press

Double Element WOD #102
21 - 15 - 9
Wall balls
OH press

Double Element WOD #103
21 - 15 - 9
Wall balls
OH squat

Double Element WOD #104
21 - 15 - 9
Wall balls
Back extensions

Double Element WOD #105
21 - 15 - 9
Wall balls
Push-ups

Double Element WOD #106
21 - 15 - 9
Wall balls
Pull-ups

Double Element WOD #107
21 - 15 - 9
Wall balls
Dips

Double Element WOD #108

21 - 15 - 9
Wall balls
Thrusters

Double Element WOD #109
21 - 15 - 9
Wall balls
Deadlift

Double Element WOD #110
21 - 15 - 9
Ring rows
Back extensions

Double Element WOD #111
21 - 15 – 9
Jumping jacks
Thrusters

Double Element WOD #112
21 - 15 – 9
Jumping jacks
OH Squats

Double Element WOD #113
21 - 15 – 9
Jumping jacks
OH Presses

Double Element WOD #114
21 - 15 – 9
Jumping jacks
Ring rows

Intermediate WODs

Intermediate WODs are the next step after your "beginner" workouts. These WODs are going to be a bit more challenging, require more equipment, and generally last a bit longer. These workouts can be scaled down or "Rx+"ed should you need an easier or more challenging workout. As with all levels of Cross Training, always start your workout with a preparation and mobility work to prevent injury, and remember to listen to your body. Make sure to challenge yourself, but if something feels like it may cause injury, then set it down and either lower your weight or scale your movement. An injury can set you back significantly in your training, so it is important to work at a level that is right for your body.

Intermediate Mixed WODs

Intermediate Mixed WOD #1
3 rounds
50x Prisoner squats
40x Sit-ups
30x Push-ups
20x Pull-ups
10x Burpees
15 ft Rope climb, 1 ascent

Intermediate Mixed WOD #2
3 rounds
21-15-9x reps
Burpees
Pull-ups
Box jumps (24 inch)
Dips

Intermediate Mixed WOD #3

2 rounds
10x Handstand push-ups
20x Burpees
30x Pull-ups
40x Pistols
50x Push-ups
10x Inverted burpees
20x Squat jumps
30x Sit-ups
40x Box jumps
50x Knees to elbows

Intermediate Mixed WOD #4
8 rounds
5x Weighted pull-ups (35#/15#)
10x Toes to bar
15x Deck squats
20x Push-ups

Intermediate Mixed WOD #5
4 rounds
40-30-20-10x reps
Burpees
Pull-ups
Squat jumps
Toes to bar
Hand release push-ups
Double-unders

Intermediate Mixed WOD #6
2 rounds
1 minute max reps pull-ups
Rest 1 minute
1 minute max reps sit-ups
Rest 1 minute

1 minute max reps box jumps (24/20")
Rest 1 minute
1 minute max reps push-ups
Rest 1 minute
1 minute max reps dips
Rest 3 minutes

Intermediate Mixed WOD #7
2 rounds
Burpee broad jumps 25m out and back
25x Pull-ups
Walking lunge 25m out and back
50x Box jumps (20 inch)
4x Sprint (25m out and back)
40x Double-unders
Bear crawl 25m out and back
20x Knees to elbows

Intermediate Mixed WOD #8
Max rounds
12 minute time cap
1x Pull-up
2x Push-ups
3x Squats
Add 1 rep to all movements each successive round, continue until failure or time elapses

Intermediate Mixed WOD #9
3 rounds
25x Squats
25x Push-ups
25x Lateral jumps over 16" obstacle
25x Sit-ups
25x Pull-ups

Run 400m

Intermediate Mixed WOD #10
For time
50x Sit-ups
50x Double unders
50x Sit-ups
50x Walking lunge steps
50x Sit-ups
50x Burpees
50x Sit-ups

Intermediate Mixed WOD #11
1 round
60x Push-ups
50x Body rows
40x Sit-ups
30x Squats
20x Dips
10x Box jumps
5x Burpees

Intermediate Mixed WOD #12
1 round
60x Push-ups
50x Body rows
40x Sit-ups
30x Squats
20x Dips
10x Box jumps
5x Burpees

Intermediate Mixed WOD #13 - Daxon
5 rounds

Run 200m
20x Pull-ups
20x Hand release push-ups
30x Sit-ups
30x Squats

Intermediate Mixed WOD #14 - Widowmaker

2 rounds
10x Handstand push-ups
20x Box jumps
30x Pull-ups
40x Push-ups
50x Double unders
10x Knees to elbows
20x Dips
30x Burpees
40x Sit-ups (feet anchored)
50x Squats

Intermediate Mixed WOD #15

5 rounds
10x Pull-ups
20x Burpees
10x Toes to bar
20x Sit-ups

Intermediate Mixed WOD #16 - No guts, no glory

3 rounds
20x Box jumps
20x Dips
20x Lunges
20x Under-the-fence push-up
20x Squats
20x Pull-ups

20x Knees to elbows
20x Burpees
20x Sit-ups
Sprint 100m (backwards on round 2)

Intermediate Mixed WOD #17
For time
50x Squats
25x Push-ups
50x Pistols
25x Fingertip push-ups
50x Jumping alternating lunges
25x knuckle push-ups
50x Walking lunges
25x Diamond push-ups

Intermediate Mixed WOD #18
For time
100x Squats
100x Pull-ups
200x Push-ups
300x Squats
100x Walking lunge steps

Intermediate Mixed WOD #19
2 rounds
35x Squats
35x Knees to elbows
35x Push-ups
35x Sit-ups
35x Pull-ups
35x Burpees
35x Double unders

Intermediate Mixed WOD #20 - Bitch better have my money

3 rounds
Run 400m
20x Pull-ups
20x Push-ups
20x Burpees
20x Squats
20x Walking lunge steps, each leg

Intermediate Mixed WOD #21

3 rounds
25x Squats
25x Push-ups
25x Lateral jumps over 16" obstacle
25x Sit-ups
25x Pull-ups
Run 400m

Intermediate Mixed WOD #22 - The Gorilla

5 rounds
15 ft Rope climb, 1 ascent
10x Pull-ups
20x Elevated sit-ups
30x Push-ups

Intermediate Mixed WOD #23 - Gizmo

3 rounds
Run 800m
10x Burpee pull-ups
20x Walking lunge steps, each leg
30x Push-ups
40x Squats
50x Double-unders

Intermediate Mixed WOD #24 - Deadbeat Dad
For time
25x Pull-ups
50x Push-ups
50x Lunges
50x Sit-ups
50x Squats
50x Flutter kicks
25x Pull-ups

Intermediate Mixed WOD #25 - Harry
3 rounds
50x Prisoner squats
40x Push ups
30x Knee to elbows
20x Burpees
10x Pull ups

Intermediate Mixed WOD #26
1 round
100x Push-ups
40x Sit-ups
30x Box jumps
20x Push-ups
10x L pull-ups
100x Burpees

Intermediate Mixed WOD #27 - Apollo
For time
50x Push-ups
50x Pull-ups
50x Hanging leg raises
50x Squats

50x Sit-ups
50x Jumping jacks

Intermediate Mixed WOD #28
For time
60x Push-ups
50x Body rows
40x Sit-ups
30x Squats
20x Dips
10x Box jumps
5x Burpees

Intermediate Mixed WOD #29
3 rounds
25x Body rows
100x Squats
35x Sit-ups
50x Jumping jacks

Intermediate Mixed WOD #30 - Tricky-Beltran
10 rounds
10-9-8-7-6-5-4-3-2-1x reps
Burpee pull-ups
Handstand push-ups
Box jumps (24 inch)

Intermediate Mixed WOD #31 - Harry
3 rounds
50x Prisoner squats
40x Push ups
30x Knee to elbows
20x Burpees

Intermediate Mixed WOD #32
2 rounds
30x Burpees
40x Overhead squat (45#)
50x Double-unders
Row 60 calories

Intermediate Mixed WOD #33
5 RFT
8x Thrusters (135#)
6x Rope climb
11x Box jumps
400m Sandbag carry

Intermediate Mixed WOD #34
3 RFT
15x Ring push-ups
10x Overhead squat (95#/65#)
10x Sumo deadlift high pull (95#/65#)
15x Lateral jumps over 20 inch obstacle

Intermediate Mixed WOD #35
5 RFT
Run 200m
10x Pull-ups
5x Power snatch (135#/95#)
Row 200m

Intermediate Mixed WOD #36
3 rounds, 21-15-9x
Knees to elbows
Turkish get-ups (40#/30# DBs)
GHD sit-ups
Back extensions

Ring push-ups

Intermediate Mixed WOD #37
6 RFT
21-18-15-12-9-6x reps
Knees to elbows
Dips (bar or rings)
Squat jumps
KB swings (53#/36#)

Intermediate Mixed WOD #38 – Junk in the Trunk
For time
25x Back squat (225#)
50x Box jump (24 inch)
75x Wall ball (20#)
100x Squats

Intermediate Mixed WOD #39
3 RFT
1-15-9x reps of
Push press (135#/95#)
Ring dips
Burpees

Intermediate Mixed WOD #40
3 RFT
Row 250m
5x Power clean (135#/95#)
10x KB swings (53#/36#)
15x Wall-ball (20#/14#)

Intermediate Mixed WOD #41 - Kickapoo
3 RFT
Row 500m

Run 400m
21x Deadlift (225#/155#)
15x Double KB jerk (53#/24#)
9x Box jumps (30/20 inch)
4x Muscle-ups

Gymnastics WODs

Gymnastics WOD #1
3 rounds
50x Squats
20x Ring push-ups
12x Pull-ups

Gymnastics WOD #2
30 rounds
2x Pistols, left leg
2x Pistols, right leg
1x Muscle-up
100m Walking lunge

Gymnastics WOD #3 - Krypto6924
10 rounds
10x Burpees
25x Squats
25x Push-ups
10x Pull-ups
10x Ring dips
25x Sit-ups

Gymnastics WOD #4
5 rounds
3x Muscle-ups

6x Forward rolls
9x Handstand push-ups
12x Pistols

Gymnastics WOD #5
3 rounds, 10-20-30x reps
Squats
Ring dips
Squats
Pull-ups
Squats

Gymnastics WOD #6
5 rounds
10x Ring dips
15x Pull-ups
20x Double unders

Gymnastics WOD #7 - Seppuku
10 rounds
10x Knees to elbows
10x Ring push-ups
10x L pull-ups

Gymnastics WOD #8
3 rounds, 10-20-30x reps
Squats
Ring dips
Squats
Pull-ups
Squats
Push-ups

Gymnastics WOD #9

5 rounds
50-40-30-20-10x
Pull-ups
Ring dips

Gymnastics WOD #10
4 rounds
50x Squats
7x Muscle-ups

Gymnastics WOD #11 - Glassman
3 rounds, 15-12-9x reps
Ring dips
Ring pull-ups
Ring Push-ups
Skin-the-cat
Muscle-ups

Gymnastics WOD #12
3 rounds
10x Handstand push-ups
15x Ring dips
20x Push-ups
45x Pull-ups

Gymnastics WOD #13
7 rounds
20x Ring dips
20x Pull-ups
20x Walking lunge steps

Gymnastics WOD #14 – Falcon Punch
10 rounds
10-9-8…3-2-1x reps

Handstand push-ups
Ring dips
Pull-ups

Rowing WODs

Rowing WOD #1
5 rounds
20x Pull-ups
30x Push-ups

Rowing WOD #2
2 rounds
Rest for exact amount of time required to complete previous interval
Row 600m
Rest
Row 1200m
Rest
Row 20000m
Rest

Rowing WOD #3
Time trial
Row 4000m

Rowing WOD #4
Intervals
Rest 2 minutes between intervals
Row 6x500m

Rowing WOD #5
Intervals

2 rounds, cover max distance
Row 1 minute
Rest 1 minute
Row 1 minute
Rest 50 seconds
Row 1 minute
Rest 40 seconds
Row 1 minute
Rest 30 seconds
Row 1 minute
Rest 20 seconds
Row 1 minute
Rest 10 seconds

Rowing WOD #6
4 rounds for max distance
Row 2 minutes
Rest 1 minute

Rowing WOD #7
Time trial
Row 8000m

Rowing WOD #8
Time trial
Row 3000m

Rowing WOD #9
Intervals
Cover max distance during each interval
Row 3 minutes
Rest 1 minute
Row 3 minutes
Rest 3 minute

Row 3 minutes
Rest 1 minute
Row 3 minutes
Rest 3 minute
Row 3 minutes

Rowing WOD #10
Intervals
Record average time for all intervals, this is an all-out effort.
Row 10x250m
Rest for 5x (interval time) after each row interval

Rowing WOD #11
Tabata
Cover max distance possible
Row 8x [20:10]

Rowing WOD #12
Intervals
Row 4x1200m
Rest 2 minutes between intervals

Rowing WOD #13
Intervals
Row 10x250m
Rest 1 minute between intervals

Rowing WOD #14
Intervals
Row 4x1200m
Rest 2 minutes between intervals

Rowing WOD #15
2 rounds

Rest for exact amount of time as previous row interval
Row 250m
Rest
Row 500m
Rest
Row 1000m
Rest
Row 2000m
Rest

Rowing WOD #16
Intervals
Row 3x2500m
Rest 1 minute between intervals

Rowing WOD #17
Intervals
Cover max distance during each interval
Row 3 minutes
Rest 2 minutes
Row 3 minutes
Rest 3 minute
Row 3 minutes
Rest 1 minute
Row 3 minutes
Rest 3 minute
Row 3 minutes
Rest 1 minute

Rowing WOD #18
Intervals
Cover max distance
Row 10x [60:60]

Rowing WOD #19
Intervals
Row 20x [15:10]

Time trial
Cover max distance
Row 10 min

Rowing WOD #20
Time trial
Cover max distance
Row 25 minutes

Rowing WOD #21
Intervals
Rest 45 seconds between intervals
Row 8x250m

Rowing WOD #22
Intervals
Cover max distance
Row 8x [30:20]

Rowing WOD #23
Intervals
Row 10x250m
Rest 1 minute between intervals

Rowing WOD #24
5 rounds
Partner effort, one rows while the other rests, switch until all rounds done
Row 50-40-30-20-10 calories

Rowing WOD #25
Time trial
Row 1500m
Damper setting at 10

Rowing WOD #26
Intervals
Record average time for all intervals
Row 10x250m
Rest for 5x (interval time)

Rowing WOD #27
3 rounds
Row 500m
Row 200m, upper body only
Rest 1 minute

Rowing WOD #28
6 rounds
Row 1000m
Rest 90 seconds

Rowing WOD #29
3 rounds
Rest for exact amount of time required to complete previous row interval
Row 250m
Rest
Row 500m
Rest
Row 750m
Rest

Rowing WOD #30

Intervals
Row 2x2500m
Rest 3 minutes between intervals

Rowing WOD #31
Rowing ladder
For total distance
Row 1 minute ON 1 minute OFF
Row 1 minute ON 50 seconds OFF
Row 1 minute ON 40 seconds OFF
Row 1 minute ON 30 seconds OFF
Continue down ladder until 1 minute ON 10 seconds OFF then back up and finish with 1 minute ON 50 seconds OFF

Rowing WOD #32
5 rounds
Rowing intervals, use total distance or calories as score
10:10
20:10
10:10
30:10:00
15:10
25:60

Rowing WOD #33
Calorie Row, 2 rounds
20:15
50:15:00
30:20:00
60:15:00
15:30
30:10:00
60:60

Rowing WOD #34
Intervals
Cover max distance
Row 6x [90:90]

Rowing WOD #35
Intervals
Rest 2 minutes between intervals
Row 6x500m

Rowing WOD #36
Intervals
Rest 45 seconds between intervals
Row 8x250m

Rowing WOD #37
3RFT
30 cal row
30 Ab mat sit-ups

Rowing WOD #38
3RFT
20 cal row
25x snatches

Rowing WOD #39
Max rounds in 15 minutes
200m row
15x Bar facing burpees
20x Push-ups

Rowing WOD #40
5RFT
300m row

20x Wall ball

Swimming WODs

Swimming WOD #1
3 rounds
Swim 25m freestyle
30x Squats
Swim 25m underwater
50x Push-ups

Swimming WOD #2
15 minute AMRAP
Swim 25m
25x Push-ups
10x KB goblet (36#/24#)

Swimming WOD #3
15 minute AMRAP
Swim 50m
2x Handstand push-ups (add 2 reps each successive round - 2, 4, 6, 8, etc.)

Swimming WOD #4
5 rounds
10x/arm KB clean & jerk (53#/36#) in shallow water
Swim 50m
Rest 1 minute

Swimming WOD #5
For time
50x Pull-ups
Swim 50m backstroke

50x Push-ups
Swim 50m butterfly
50x Sit ups
Swim 50m freestyle

Swimming WOD #6
For time/reps
Max reps unbroken handstand push-ups
Swim 50m for time
Rest 2 minutes
Max reps unbroken push-ups
Swim 50m for time
Rest 2 minutes
Max reps unbroken pull-ups
Swim 50m for time

Swimming WOD #7
5 rounds
Underwater swim 25m
50x Squats

Swimming WOD #8
3 rounds
Swim 200m
30x KB swings (53#/36#)
30x Pull-ups or body rows

Swimming WOD #9
For max reps
Tread water 3 minutes
1 minute push-ups
Tread water 2 minutes
1 minute sit-ups
Tread water 1 minute

1 minute squats

Swimming WOD #10
3 rounds
Swim 50m
15x Deadlift (225#/185#)
30x Double-unders

Swimming WOD #11
7 rounds
100m freestyle
50x Squats
Rest 2 minutes

Swimming WOD #12
2 rounds
20x Man-makers (50#/35# DBs)
Swim 100m
10x/arm KB snatch (53#/36#)
Swim 100m
20x Deadlift (185#/135#)

Swimming WOD #13
For time
Swim 200m
Then,
21-15-9x reps of
Push-press (115#/80#)
KB swing (53#/36#)
Then,
Finish with 200m swim

Swimming WOD #14
Max rounds in 10 minutes

Swim 50m
10x Burpees
15x Squats

Swimming WOD #15
3 rounds
Swim 50m
15x Deadlift (225#/185#)
30x Box jumps

Swimming WOD #16
For time
Swim 50m
50x Squats
Swim 50m, pull only
50x Sit-ups
Swim 50m, kick only
50x Push-ups
Swim 50m

Swimming WOD #17
Max rounds in 15 minutes
Swim 25m
9x HSPU
10x KB goblet (36#/24#)

Swimming WOD #18
4 rounds
Swim 25m
Walking lunges 25m
Swim 25m underwater
Bear crawl 25m
Rest 1 minute

Swimming WOD #19
3 rounds
Swim 25m
25x Push-ups
Swim 25m underwater
5x Snatches
10x Burpees

Swimming WOD #20
For time
200m Underwater dolphin kick with fins
50m KB farmers carry underwater (2x53#/36#)
100x Double-unders
50m KB farmers carry underwater
Swim 100m freestyle
Swim 100m backstroke

Swimming WOD #21
3 rounds
Swim 25m backstroke
Swim 25m underwater
15x Deadlift (185#/135#)
30x Push-ups

Swimming WOD #22
For time
50m Single KB farmers carry poolside (72#/53#)
Swim 50m
100m Farmers Carry
Swim 100m
150m Farmers Carry
Swim 200m

Swimming WOD #23

8 rounds
25m Farmers carry underwater (2x53#/36#)
25m Farmers carry poolside

Swimming WOD #24
3 rounds
Wearing fins and snorkel
Swim 200m
35x Squats
25x Push-ups
20x Sit-ups

Swimming WOD #25
10 rounds
Swim 50m any style
25x Push-ups

Swimming WOD #26
10 rounds
Swim 50m any style
25x Sit-ups

Swimming WOD #27
10 rounds
Swim 50m any style
25x Back extension

Swimming WOD #28
For total time
Swim 1000m
Rest 5 minutes
Then, 3 rounds of
25x Thruster (45#/30# DBs)
Swim 50m

Swimming WOD #29
3 rounds
21x Deadlift (225#/185#)
Swim 200m
Rest 3 minutes

Swimming WOD #30
3 rounds
15x OH Squats
Swim 500m
Rest 3 minutes

Swimming WOD #31
5 rounds
10x Thrusters
Swim 300m
Rest 3 minutes

Kettlebell WODs

Kettlebell WOD #1
8 RFT
50x SU jump rope
15x KB swing

Kettlebell WOD #2
10 RFT
35x DU jump rope
30x KB swing

Kettlebell WOD #3
20 minute AMRAP

50x SU jump rope
15x KB swings
20x walking lunge with KB

Kettlebell WOD #4
15 minute AMRAP
30x DU jump rope
30x walking lunge with KB
30x KB swings

Kettlebell WOD #5
Double Handed Kettlebell Swing – 30 secs
Rest 30 seconds
Repeat 5-10 times

Kettlebell WOD #6
Single Handed Kettlebell Swing – 20 reps each side
Turkish Get Ups – 1 each side
Rest 1-2 minutes
Repeat adding 1 extra Turkish Get Up
Stop when your Turkish Get Ups begin to lose form

Kettlebell WOD #7
Single Handed Swing – 20 reps each side
Push Ups – 10 reps
Repeat 5-10 times

Kettlebell WOD #8
5 minute AMRAP
5 double kettlebell thruster (if you have lower back/mobility issues you could perform a push press with a bigger dip)
5 double kettlebell cleans
5 double kettlebell swings
6 Box jumps step down

Kettlebell WOD #9
4 minute AMRAP
4 double kettlebell thruster
4 double kettlebell cleans
4 double kettlebell swings
5 Box jumps step down

Kettlebell WOD #10
3 minute AMRAP
3 double kettlebell thruster
3 double kettlebell cleans
3 double kettlebell swings
4 box jumps step down

Kettlebell WOD #11
For time
100x KB squat clean to thruster (72#/53#)
Use a single KB, switch hands every rep

Kettlebell WOD #12
1 round
Row 2000m
200x KB swings (72#/53#)
Row 2000m

Kettlebell WOD #13
Max reps in 10 minutes
Switch arms as necessary, KB may not touch floor
Long cycle KB clean & jerk (53#/36#)

Kettlebell WOD #14
3 rounds
1 minute snatch AMRAP each arm

Rest 2 minutes between rounds
3 rounds
1 minute double kettlebell jerk
Rest 2 minutes between rounds
3 rounds
1 minute goblet squat

Kettlebell WOD #15
4 RFT
15 double-arm swings
10 Goblet squats

Kettlebell WOD #16
Run 200m
100 single-arm swings (50/50)
50 burpees (sub light goblet squats for burpees if needed)
Run 200m
75 double-arm swings (heavier than your single arm weight)
25 Burpees
Run 200m
50 single-arm swings (25/25)
15 Burpees
Run 200m

Kettlebell WOD #17
10 Swings
Goblet Squat 1 rep
15 Swings
Goblet Squat 2 reps
25 Swings
Goblet Squat 3 reps
50 Swings
Rest 30-60 seconds; repeat 4 more times.

Kettlebell WOD #18

10 Swings
Dip 2 reps
15 Swings
Dip 3 reps
25 Swings
Dip 5 reps
50 Swings
Rest 30-60 seconds; repeat 4 more times.

Kettlebell WOD #19

10 Swings
Press 1 rep (double kettlebell press)
15 Swings
Press 2 reps
25 Swings
Press 3 reps
50 Swings
Rest 30-60 seconds; repeat 4 more times.

Kettlebell WOD #20

10 Swings
Chin-up 1 rep
15 Swings
Chin-up 2 reps
25 Swings
Chin-up 3 reps
50 Swings
Rest 30-60 seconds; repeat 4 more times.

Kettlebell WOD #21

3 rounds
6x KB turkish get-up (53#/24#)
6x KB clean/press/windmill combo (36#/18#)

50m Heavy sandbag carry

Kettlebell WOD #22
3 rounds
30x Double KB swings (53#/36#)
25x Chest to bar pull-ups
20x Double KB shoulder to overhead (53#/36#)

Kettlebell WOD #23
15 rounds
KB snatch (53#) 1-2-3-4...13-14-15x reps, switch arms each round
Push-ups 15-14-13-12...3-2-1x reps

Kettlebell WOD #24
3 rounds
21-15-9x reps
Bottoms-up KB thruster (72#)
Box jump
Burpee broad jumps

Kettlebell WOD #25
For time
400m KB Farmer's walk (2x53#)
50x Bottoms-up single KB thruster (53#)
25x/arm KB snatch
50x Alternating floor press
400m KB Farmer's walk

Kettlebell WOD #26
3 rounds
9x KB suitcase deadlift (2x88#)
12x/arm KB snatch (53#)
15x KB push press (2x44#)

Kettlebell WOD #27 - Ratchet #3
18 rounds
1-2-3-2-3-4-3-4-5-4-5-6-5-6-7-6-7-8x reps
Push-press (2x53#)
Bent row

Kettlebell WOD #28
29 rounds
Breathing ladder
KB swing (53#) 1-15-1

Kettlebell WOD #29
5 rounds
30x ring rows
8x KB swings (106#/72#)
10x KB press, each arm (53#/24#)
12x Knees to elbows

Kettlebell WOD #30
5 rounds
Sprint 50m
35x KB Swings (53#)
30x KB walking Lunges (2x36#)
25x Sit-ups

Kettlebell WOD #31
EMOM for 16 minutes
8x KB swings (72#/53#)
3x Double KB jerk (2x53#/36#)

Dumbbell WODs

Dumbbell WOD #1
For time
50x Single dumbbell snatch

Dumbbell WOD #2
For time
100x Single dumbbell snatch

Dumbbell WOD #3
For time
50x Single dumbbell hang snatch

Dumbbell WOD #4
For time
100x Single dumbbell hang snatch

Dumbbell WOD #5
For time
50x Double dumbbell clean

Dumbbell WOD #6
For time
100x Double dumbbell clean

Dumbbell WOD #7
For time
50x Clean and Jerk with dumbbells

Dumbbell WOD #8
For time
100x Clean and Jerks with dumbbells

Dumbbell WOD #9
For time

50x 3 position Clean and 1 Jerk with dumbbells

Dumbbell WOD #10
For time
50x Hang Clean and Jerk with dumbbells

Dumbbell WOD #11
For time
100x Hang Clean and Jerk with dumbbells

Dumbbell WOD #12
For time
50x Overhead Squat with dumbbells

Dumbbell WOD #13
For time
100x Overhead Squat with dumbbells

Dumbbell WOD #14
For time
50x Strict press with dumbbells

Dumbbell WOD #15
For time
100x Strict press with dumbbells

Dumbbell WOD #16
For time
50x Push Press with dumbbells

Dumbbell WOD #17
For time
100x Push Press with dumbbells

Dumbbell WOD #18
For time
50x Double dumbbell lift

Dumbbell WOD #19
For time
100x Double dumbbell lift

Dumbbell WOD #20
For time
75x SDHP with dumbbells

Dumbbell WOD #21
For time
50x Chest Press with dumbbells

Dumbbell WOD #22
For time
100x Chest Press with dumbbells

Dumbbell WOD #23
Max Rounds in 20 minutes
Each round 50x Bench Press
2 minute rest in between

Dumbbell WOD #24
For time
50x Thrusters with dumbbells

Dumbbell WOD #25
For time
100x Thrusters with dumbbells

Dumbbell WOD #26

5 RFT
30x Dumbbell Swings

Dumbbell WOD #27
3 RFT
35 pound Dumbbell squat snatch, 15 reps, right arm
15 GHD sit-ups
35 pound Dumbbell squat snatch, 15 reps, left arm
15 Toes to bar

Dumbbell WOD #28
21-15-9
Thruster w/45# dumbbells
Burpee
Immediately after: Sprint at the highest incline and the fastest speed you can handle for 2 minutes. Increase the speed as you go.

Dumbbell WOD #29
100 db push press @ 45# dumbbells
At the start of every minute perform 3 burpees until you finish

Dumbbell WOD #30
Every minute on the minute:
10 thrusters @ 40# db's
20 double unders

Dumbbell WOD #31
5 rounds:
Run 400 meters
20 Hang Squat Cleans @ 35# dumbbells
15 burpees

Dumbbell WOD #32

100 hang squat clean thrusters w/ 35# dumbbells
At the start of every minute perform 5 burpees

Dumbbell WOD #33
Run for 5 minutes at a moderate pace on the treadmill.
At minute 6 perform max snatches in 2 minutes alternating arms with the dumbbell.
At minute 9 perform max KB swings w/dumbbell in 1 minute
At minute 11 perform max front squats holding the same dumbbell for 2 minutes
At minute 14 perform max burpees for 1 minute

Dumbbell WOD #34
3 Wall Climbs (walk your feet up a wall while facing the wall, walk back down...may want to do it outside)
7 squat cleans w/45# dumbbells

Dumbbell WOD #35
AMRAP 10 minutes:
10 Push Press w/35# dumbbells
5 burpees

Benchmark WODs

Benchmark WOD #1 – Barbara
5 rounds
20x Pull-ups
30x Push-ups
40x Sit-ups
50x Squats
10x Sit-ups
10x Prisoner squats

Benchmark WOD #2 - Mila
For time
30x Pull-ups, kipping
Run 400m
12x Pull-ups, strict
Run 400m
5x Pull-ups, weighted (35#/20#)
Run 400m

Benchmark WOD #3 - Mel
5 rounds
Run 100m
10x Burpees
10x Push-ups
10x Mountain climbers

Benchmark WOD #4 – Annie
5 rounds, 50-40-30-20-10x reps
Double unders
Sit-ups

Benchmark WOD #5 – Mary
Max rounds in 20 minutes
5x Handstand push-ups
10x Pistols
15x Pull-ups

Benchmark WOD #6 – Susan
5 rounds
Run 200m
10x Push-ups
10x Squats

Benchmark WOD #7 - The other Lynn

Max rounds in 20 minutes
25x Squats
20x Push-ups
15x Box jumps (24 inch)
10x Burpees
5x Pull-ups

Benchmark WOD #8 – Taylor
4 rounds
3x Back walk-overs
10m Handstand walk
20x Knees to elbows

Benchmark WOD #9 - Grace
For time
30x Clean & jerk (135#)

Benchmark WOD #10 - Nicole
Max rounds in 20 minutes
Run 400m
Max rep pull-ups

Benchmark WOD #11 - Angie
For time
100x Pull-ups
100x Push-ups
100x Sit-ups
100x Squats

Benchmark WOD #12 - Amanda
3 rounds
9-7-5x
Muscle-up
Snatch (135#/95#)

Benchmark WOD #13 – Kelly
5 rounds
Run 400m
30x Box jump (24 inch)
30x Wall ball (20#)

Benchmark WOD #14 - Elizabeth
3 rounds
21-15-9x reps
Clean (135#)
Ring dips

Benchmark WOD #15 - Karen
For time
150x Wall ball (20#)

Benchmark WOD #16 - Isabel
For time
30x Snatch (135#)

Benchmark WOD #17 – Eva
5 rounds
Run 800m
30x KB swing (72#)
30x Pull-ups

Benchmark WOD #18 - Jackie
For time
Row 1000m
50x Thruster (45#)
30x Pull-ups

Benchmark WOD #19 - Diane

3 rounds
21-15-9x reps
Deadlift (225#)
Handstand push-ups

Benchmark WOD #20 - Nancy

5 rounds
Run 400m
15x Overhead squat (95#)

Benchmark WOD #21 - Linda

10 rounds
10-9-8-7-6-5-4-3-2-1x
Deadlift (1 1/2 bw)
Bench Press (bw)
Clean (3/4 bw)

Benchmark WOD #22 - Nasty Girls 2.0

3 rounds
50x Pistol squats, alternating
7x Muscle-ups
10x Hang power clean (175#)

Benchmark WOD #23 – Fran

3 rounds
21-15-9x reps
Thruster (95#)
Pull-ups

Benchmark WOD #24 – Helen

3 rounds
Run 400m
21x KB swing (53#)
12x Pull-ups

Benchmark WOD #25 - Lynne
5 rounds for max reps
Bench press (bw)
Pull-ups

Benchmark WOD #26 - Chelsea
Top of each minute for 30 minutes
5x Pull-ups
10x Push-ups
15x Squats

Benchmark WOD #27 - Cindy
20 minute AMRAP
5 Pull-ups
10 Push-ups
15 Squats

EMOM (Every minute on the minute) WODs

EMOM WOD #1
EMOM for 5 minutes
1x Clean & jerk (95% 1RM)
Rest 1 minute
1 minute max reps deadlift (75% 1RM)
Rest 1 minute
Repeat EMOM 5: 3x C&J (80% 1RM)

EMOM WOD #2
EMOM for 8 minutes
3x Cluster (185#/135#)
7x Burpees

EMOM WOD #3
EMOM for 20 minutes
First minute - 3x Push press (as heavy as possible)
Second minute - 3x Back squat (as heavy as possible)

EMOM WOD #4
EMOM for 12 minutes
1x Power clean (95% 1RM)
3x Chest to bar pull-ups
Sprint 20m out and back

EMOM WOD #5
EMOM for 12 minutes
1x Deadlift (315#/205#)
3x Burpees
5x KB swings (72#/53#)

EMOM WOD #6
EMOM for 10 minutes
5x Deadlift (315#/225#)
5x Shoulder to overhead (185#/135#)

EMOM WOD #7
EMOM for max rounds
2x Back squat (135#/75#)
Add 10# per minute up to 225#/135#
After that add 5# each additional minute until failure

EMOM WOD #8
EMOM for 10 minutes
3x Back squat (275#/185#)
Prowler/sled push, 20 yds out and back (AHAP)

EMOM WOD #9

EMOM for 30 minutes
2x Cluster (185#/135#)

EMOM WOD #10
EMOM for 20 minutes
Set up two barbells...
First minute - 5x Hang snatch (start at 50% 1RM, add some weight as you continue)
Second minute - 2x Front squat + 1x Shoulder to overhead (use 70-80% C&J 1RM)

EMOM WOD #11
EMOM for 10 minutes
5x Dips
4x Pull-ups
3x Handstand push-ups

EMOM WOD #12
EMOM for 10 minutes
2x Clean and jerk (3RM)
7x Toes to bar

EMOM WOD #13
EMOM for max rounds
1x Bench press (bw)
1x Burpee
Add 1 rep every minute thereafter and continue until failure

EMOM WOD #14
EMOM for 12 minutes
5x Ground to overhead (135#/115#)
15x Push-ups

EMOM WOD #15

EMOM for 10 minutes
3x Deadlift (375#/275#)
5x Box jumps (36/30 inch)

EMOM WOD #16
EMOM
Add 2x reps per round, continue until failure
2x Back squat (185#/95#)

EMOM WOD #17
Every 4 minutes on the minute for 24 minutes
Run 400m
12x Burpee box jump-overs (24/20")
(6 rounds total)

EMOM WOD #18
Every 4 minutes on the minute for 24 minutes
Run 400m
12x Burpee box jump-overs (24/20")
(6 rounds total)

EMOM WOD #19
EMOM for 12 minutes
2x Deadlift (315#/205#)
5x Burpees
9x KB swings (72#/53#)

EMOM WOD #20
EMOM for 24 minutes
First minute - 30x Double-unders
Second minute - 20x Burpees
Third minute - 15x KB swings (53#/36#)

EMOM WOD #21

EMOM for 16 minutes
5x Burpees
15x Double unders

EMOM WOD #22
Every second minute on the minute for max rounds
10x Overhead squat (95#/65#)
10x Chest-to-bar pull-ups

Add 2 reps per round until you can no longer perform the requisite number of reps within the two minute period.

EMOM WOD #23
EMOM for 15 minutes
First minute: 7x Push press (155#/115#)
Second minute: 20x KB swings (72#/53#)
Third minute: 40x Double-unders
Repeat triplet for 15 minutes

EMOM WOD #24
EMOM for 16 minutes
Odd minutes: 6x Front squat (135#/95#) + 6x Burpee over bar
Even minutes: 30 seconds row for max calories (start at 0:15 into minute, finish at 0:45)

EMOM WOD #25
EMOM for 10 minutes
50 ft Farmers walk (100# per hand)
3x Ground to shoulder (bw)

EMOM WOD #26
EMOM for 12 minutes
1x Power clean (95% 1RM)
3x Chest to bar pull-ups

Sprint 20m out and back

EMOM WOD #27
EMOM for max rounds
1x Bench press (bw)
1x Burpee
Add 1 rep every minute thereafter and continue until failure

EMOM WOD #28
EMOM for max rounds
3x Back squat (80% 1RM)
5x Strict pull-ups
sprint 40 yards
Each minute thereafter add 1 rep to the squat, continue until failure.

EMOM WOD #29
EMOM for 30 minutes
First minute: 4x Front squats (1.3x bw)
Second minute: 3x Stone to shoulder (bw)
Third minute: 4x Bench press (1.3x bw)

EMOM WOD #30
EMOM for 20 minutes
5x Back squats (5RM) - even minutes
3x Power clean (3RM) - odd minutes

EMOM WOD #31
EMOM for 15 minutes
1x Deadlift (155#/105#)
1x Hang power clean
1x Front squat
1x Push press

EMOM WOD #32
EMOM for 18 Mins
10 Deadlift @ 50% 1RM
5 Box Jumps

EMOM WOD #33
EMOM for 14 Mins
3 Broad Jumps
15 metre Bear Crawl
5 V-Ups

EMOM WOD #34
EMOM for 14 Mins
5 Air Squats
5 Sit Ups
3 Broad Jumps

EMOM WOD #35
EMOM for 18 Mins
2 Clean & Jerk @ 70% 1RM
5 Broad Jumps

EMOM WOD #36
For Time
100 KB Swings
EMOM perform 5 box jumps

Perform 100 kettlebell swings for time. Every minute on the minute complete 5 box jumps until the 100 kb swings are complete.

EMOM WOD #37
EMOM for 14 Mins
3 Burpees

15 metre Bear Crawl
5 V-Ups

EMOM WOD #38
EMOM for 14 Mins
5 Air Squats
2 Pistols Each Side
10 Hip Bridge Extensions

EMOM WOD #39
EMOM for 14 Mins
5 Air Squats
6 Jumping Lunges (Alternating Legs)
5 Hollow Rocks

EMOM WOD #40
EMOM for 15 Mins
10 Pull-ups
5 Burpees
10 Thrusters

AMRAP WODs

AMRAP WOD #1
Max rounds in 4 minutes
2x Bench press (225#/135#)
5x Strict pull-ups
1x 20m shuttle run
Rest 2:00 between rounds, repeat for a total of 4 rounds

AMRAP WOD #2
Max rounds in 5 minutes
4x Thruster (155#)

4x Box jumps (30 inch)
Rest 2 minutes after last rep, repeat for a second round

AMRAP WOD #3
Max rounds in 6 minutes
8x Thrusters (155#)
12x Box jumps (36 inch + 20# vest)

AMRAP WOD #4
Max rounds in 6 minutes
3x Power clean (155#+)
6x Push-ups
9x Ring dips
Row 12 calories
Rest 3 minutes, repeat for 3 rounds total

AMRAP WOD #5
Max rounds in 6 minutes
3x Deadlift (135#/95#)
3x Hang power clean
3x Push press
3x Muscle-ups
20 Double-unders
Rest 2:00 after last rep, repeat AMRAP for 3 rounds total

AMRAP WOD #6
Max rounds in 6 minutes
8x Thrusters (155#)
12x Box jumps (36 inch + 20# vest)

AMRAP WOD #7 - Broken Burpees
Max rounds in 7 minutes
7x Push-ups
7x Sprawl

7x Squat jumps

AMRAP WOD #8
Max rounds in 7 minutes
5x Handstand push-ups
5x Deadlift (315#/225#)

AMRAP WOD #9
Max rounds in 7 minutes
2x Deadlift (405#/295#)
5x Handstand push-ups

AMRAP WOD #10
Max rounds in 8 minutes
1x Deadlift (365#)
3x Squat clean (225#)
5x Push jerk (165#)
15 ft Rope climb, 1 ascent

AMRAP WOD #11
Max rounds in 8 minutes
Row 200m
8x KB swing (72#/53#)
5x Pull-ups

AMRAP WOD #12
Max rounds in 8 minutes
4x Handstand push-ups on paralettes
8x KB swings (72#)
12x GHD sit-ups

AMRAP WOD #13
Max rounds in 8 minutes
4x Handstand push-ups

8x KB swings (72#)
12x Knees to elbows

AMRAP WOD #14 – Gambit
Max rounds in 8 minutes
2x Hang power clean (225#)
3x Bench press (275#)
4x Back squat (315#)
5x Deadlift (365#)

AMRAP WOD #15
Max rounds in 8 minutes
3x Overhead squat (80-85% 1RM)
3x Deadlift (90-95% 1RM)
5x Muscle-ups

AMRAP WOD #16
Max rounds in 8 minutes
1x Deadlift (1RM)
2x Muscle-up
3x Squat clean (80% 1RM)
4x Handstand push-ups

AMRAP WOD #17
Max rounds in 8 minutes
5x Overhead squat (60% 1RM)
30x Push-ups

AMRAP WOD #18
Max rounds in 8 minutes
Row 250m
5x Deadlift (315#/225#)
5x Jerk (205#/135#)

AMRAP WOD #19
Max rounds in 8 minutes
5x Squat clean (275#/155#)
9x Close-grip bench press (225#/135#)

AMRAP WOD #20
Max rounds in 8 minutes
7x Thruster (115#)
10x Sumo deadlift high pull (115#)

AMRAP WOD #21
Max rounds in 8 minutes
3x Power clean (265#/165#)
7x/arm single KB thruster (72#/53#)

AMRAP WOD #22
Max rounds in 9 minutes
3x Front squat (5RM)
3x Bench press (5RM)
3x Deadlift (5RM)

AMRAP WOD #23
2x [Max rounds in 10 minutes]
5x Handstand push-ups
20x Box jumps (20 inch)
Then,
5x Pull-ups
10x/arm KB snatch (36#)

AMRAP WOD #24
Max rounds in 10 minutes
6x Squat clean (135#/95#)
12x Pull-ups
15x Double unders

AMRAP WOD #25
Max rounds in 10 minutes
5x/arm DB Turkish get-ups (40#/25#)
15x Double-unders
20x Sit-ups

AMRAP WOD #26
Max rounds in 10 minutes
5x Thruster (135#/95#)
7x Chest to bar pull-ups
25x Double-unders

AMRAP WOD #27
Max rounds in 10 minutes
6x Sandbag Turkish get-up (100#)
6x KB swing (106#)

AMRAP WOD #28
Max rounds in 10 minutes
10x Burpee box jumps (20 inch)
10x Squat clean (155#/115#)

AMRAP WOD #29
Max rounds in 10 minutes
5x Ground to overhead (255#/155#)
KB farmer's carry, 25m out and back (88#/53#)

AMRAP WOD #30
Max rounds in 10 minutes
15x KB Swing (72#/53#)
10x Handstand push-ups
10x Double KB swing (2x53#/36#)
3x Muscle-up

AMRAP WOD #31
Max rounds in 10 minutes
Sprint 25m out and back
9x Deadlift (315#/225#)
6x Burpee bar muscle-ups

AMRAP WOD #32
Max rounds in 12 minutes
2x Squat clean (225#/135#)
4x Handstand push-ups
6x Chest to bar pull-ups

AMRAP WOD #33
Max rounds in 12 minutes
3x Thruster (135#/95#)
5x Weighted pull-ups (35#/20#)

AMRAP WOD #34
Max rounds in 12 minutes
1x Power snatch (115#/80#)
2x GHD sit-ups
3x Ring dips
Add 2 reps per movement each successive round

AMRAP WOD #35
Max rounds in 12 minutes
Row 250m
5x Thrusters (135#/95#)
10x Burpee box jump (24/20 inch)
5x Handstand push-up

AMRAP WOD #36
Max rounds in 12 minutes

7x Handstand push-ups
12x L pull-ups

AMRAP WOD #37 – Izzy
Max rounds in 12 minutes
3x/arm KB snatch (53#/36#)
5x Burpees
7x Box jumps (20/16 inch)

AMRAP WOD #38
Max rounds in 12 minutes
Row 250m
12x Ball slams (30#/20#)
6x Burpees

AMRAP WOD #39
Max rounds in 12 minutes
5x Push-press (95#/65#)
10x KB swings (53#/36#)
15x Squats

AMRAP WOD #40
Max rounds in 12 minutes
7x DB thrusters (50#+)
7x Ball slams (40#+)
Row 250m

AMRAP WOD #41
Max rounds in 12 minutes
15x KB swing (72#/53#)
5x/side Single KB thruster (53#/36#)
30x Double-unders

AMRAP WOD #42

Max rounds in 12 minutes
5x Pull-ups
10x Push-ups
15x Squats
20 cal row

AMRAP WOD #43
Max rounds in 12 minutes
5x Double KB snatch (AHAP)
5x Strict pull-ups
5x Handstand push-ups

AMRAP WOD #44
Max rounds in 13 minutes
Row 20 calories
30x Double-unders
40x KB swings (53#/36#)

AMRAP WOD #45 – 15.3
Max rounds in 14 minutes
7x Muscle-ups
50x Wall ball (20#)
100x Double-unders

AMRAP WOD #46
Max rounds in 14 minutes
10x Wall ball (20#/14#)
10x Hang power snatch (75#/55#)
25x Double-unders

AMRAP WOD #47
Max rounds in 15 minutes
3x Thruster (95#/65#)
6x Box jump (24/20 inch)

9x KB swings (53#/36#)

AMRAP WOD #48
Max rounds in 15 minutes
5x Thrusters (95#/65#)
10x Kettlebell Swings (53#/36#)
15x Burpees

AMRAP WOD #49
Max rounds in 15 minutes
Use heaviest sandbag possible
2x Turkish get-up
10x Zercher squat
12x Lateral hops over bag

AMRAP WOD #50
Max rounds in 15 minutes
15x Box jumps (24/20")
12x Push press (115#/75#)
9x Toes to bar

AMRAP WOD #51
Max rounds in 15 minutes
7x Hang squat clean (155#/110#)
20x Pull-ups
9x Box jumps (24/20 inch)

AMRAP WOD #52
Max rounds in 15 minutes
3x Muscle-ups
5x Ground to overhead (135#/95#)
7x Box jumps (24/20")
Row 200m

AMRAP WOD #53 - The Incredible Shrinking Bear

Max rounds in 15 minutes
5x Deadlift
5x Hang power clean
5x Front squat
5x Push press
5x Back squat

From 0:00 to 4:59 working load is 155#/105#
From 5:00 to 9:59 working load is 135#/85#
From 10:00 to 15:00 working load is 115#/65#

AMRAP WOD #54

Max rounds in 15 minutes
15x Double unders
10x KB swings (72#)
5x Pull-ups

AMRAP WOD #55

Max rounds in 15 minutes
15x Box jumps (24/20")
12x Push press (115#/75#)
9x Toes to bar

AMRAP WOD #56

Max rounds in 15 minutes
5x Overhead press, anyhow (185#)
10x Push-ups
15x GHD back extensions

AMRAP WOD #57

Max rounds in 15 minutes
3x Handstand push-ups
6x Pull-ups, strict

9x Knees to elbows

AMRAP WOD #58
Max rounds in 15 minutes
30x Burpees
40x Overhead squat (45#)
50x Double-unders
60 cal row

AMRAP WOD #59 - Eat The Bear
Max rounds in 15 minutes
15x KB swings
50 ft Bear crawl (25 out and back)
10x Burpees
50 ft Bear crawl
2x Wall climb

AMRAP WOD #60
Max rounds in 15 minutes
10x Deadlifts (185#)
10x Ring dips

AMRAP WOD #61
Max rounds in 15 minutes
7x Clean & jerk (135#/95#)
20x Toes to bar

AMRAP WOD #62
Max rounds in 15 minutes
5x Snatch grip deadlift (1/2 bw)
5x Hang power snatch
5x Overhead squats
5x Behind neck push jerk, snatch grip

AMRAP WOD #63
Max rounds in 15 minutes
7x Push press (135#)
10x Overhead squats (135#)
15x GHD sit-ups

AMRAP WOD #64
Max rounds in 15 minutes
10x Handstand push-ups
20x Target burpees, 6" above reach
Row 30 calories

AMRAP WOD #65
Max rounds in 15 minutes
10x Muscle-ups
10x Pistol squats
50x Double-unders

AMRAP WOD #66 - Inside-out Bear Complex
Max rounds in 15 minutes
7x Power clean (135#/95#)
7x Push press
7x Back squat

Dropping the bar at any time during a round is a 10 burpee penalty

AMRAP WOD #67 - AMRAP Party!
8 minute AMRAP
40x Double-unders
30x Wall ball (20#/14#)
Row 20 calories
- Rest 3 minutes -
Max rounds in 5 minutes

30x Double-unders
20x Wall ball (30#/20#)
- Rest 3 minutes -
Max rounds in 3 minutes
15x Double-unders
Row 10 calories

AMRAP WOD #68 – Crazy 8s

Max rounds in 18 minutes
8x Power clean (95#/70#)
8x Front squat
8x Pendlay row
8x Sumo deadlift high-pulls
8x Push press
8x Stiff-leg deadlift
8x/leg Lunges
8x Thruster

AMRAP WOD #69

Max rounds in 18 minutes
Sled push 20-yards out and back (as heavy as possible)
18x Box jumps (24/20")
16x Ball slams (20/12)
14x Renegade rows (35#/20# DBs)

AMRAP WOD #70

Max rounds in 20 minutes
15x Pull-ups
10x Pistols
5x Handstand push-ups

AMRAP WOD #71

Max rounds in 20 minutes
5x Chest to bar pull-ups

10x Wall ball (20#/14#)
15x KB swings (53#/36#)

AMRAP WOD #72
Max rounds in 20 minutes
15x Overhead squats (95#/65#)
10x Knees to elbows
5x Handstand push-ups

AMRAP WOD #73
Max rounds in 20 minutes
7x Back squat (185#)
DB overhead walking lunge, 10 steps (45# right hand)
7x Burpees
DB overhead walking lunge, 10 steps (left hand)

AMRAP WOD #74
Max rounds in 20 minutes
15x KB swings (53#/36#)
15x Push-ups
15x Pull-ups
15x KB goblet squats

AMRAP WOD #75
Max rounds in 20 minutes
12x Power snatch (75#/55#)
10x Push-ups
4x Box jumps (20 inch)

AMRAP WOD #76
Max rounds in 20 minutes
5x Double KB front squat (2x53#/36#)
10x Wall ball (20#/14#)
15x KB swings (72#/53#)

AMRAP WOD #77
Max rounds in 20 minutes
15x Wall ball (20#/14#)
10x Deadlifts (135#/95#)
5x Ring dips

AMRAP WOD #78
Max rounds in 20 minutes
3x Squat clean (135#/85#)
5x Thruster
7x Back squat
9x Push press
Run 200m

AMRAP WOD #79
Max rounds in 20 minutes
3x Deadlift (60% bw)
3x Hang clean
3x Front-squat
3x Shoulder to overhead

AMRAP WOD #80 - Buck Furpees
Max rounds in 20 minutes
5x Thruster (95#/75#)
10x Pull-ups
15x Burpees

AMRAP WOD #81
Max rounds in 20 minutes
10x Pull-ups
7x Overhead squats (95#/65#)
5x Ring dips

AMRAP WOD #82
Max rounds in 20 minutes
4x Overhead squat (135#/95#)
6x Clean & Jerk (155#/115#)
8x Toes to bar
10x Sit-ups

AMRAP WOD #83
Max rounds in 20 minutes
1x Snatch (155#/95#)
2x Muscle-ups
3x Overhead squats (155#/95)
4x Pull-ups (chest to bar)

AMRAP WOD #84
Max rounds in 20 minutes
15x Squats
10x Push-ups
5x Pull-ups

AMRAP WOD #85 - Tribute To Jack
Max rounds in 20 minutes
10x Thruster (115#)
10x KB swing (53#)
10x Burpees

AMRAP WOD #86
Max rounds in 20 minutes
10x Burpee over 16" obstacle
30x Squats
60-second handstand hold

AMRAP WOD #87 - Medicine ball Makimba
Max rounds in 20 minutes

1 round = entire Makimba WOD holding 20#/14# medicine ball
15x Thruster
10x Burpee
5x Squat

AMRAP WOD #88 – TK
Max rounds in 20 minutes
8x Strict Pull-ups
8x Box jumps (36 inch)
12x KB swings (72#)

AMRAP WOD #89
Max rounds in 20 minutes
25x Burpees
15x Back squat (bw)

AMRAP WOD #90
Max rounds in 20 minutes
12x Power snatch (75#/55#)
10x Push-ups
4x Box jumps (20 inch)

AMRAP WOD #91 - Nick Special
Max rounds in 20 minutes
10x Sumo deadlift high pull (95#)
10x Burpees
10x KB swings (72#)
10x Thrusters (95#)

AMRAP WOD #92 - Increased Gravity
Max rounds in 20 minutes
20x Burpees
5x Pull-ups

10x KB swings (53#)
20x Sit-ups

AMRAP WOD #93 - A B*tch Named Cindy
Max rounds in 20 minutes
5x Muscle-ups
10x Ring push-ups
15x Squat jumps

AMRAP WOD #94
Max rounds in 20 minutes
10x Burpees
20x Front squats
30x Double unders

AMRAP WOD #95
Max rounds in 20 minutes
5x Burpee-pull ups
7x Ring push-ups
9x Front squat (95#/75#)

AMRAP WOD #96
Max rounds in 20 minutes
Run 200m
10x Strict pull-ups
10x Clapping push-ups
25x Squats

AMRAP WOD #97 – Foo
Max rounds in 20 minutes
Start with 13x bench press (170#)
Then,
Max rounds in 20 minutes of
7x Chest to bar pull-ups

77x Double-unders
2x Squat clean thruster (aka. "cluster") (170#)
28x Sit-ups

AMRAP WOD #98

Max rounds in 20 minutes
Run 200m
10x Handstand push-ups
30x Push-ups
25x Double-unders

AMRAP WOD #99

Max rounds in 20 minutes
3x Deadlift (60% bw)
3x Hang clean
3x Front-squat
3x Shoulder to overhead

AMRAP WOD #100

Max rounds in 15 minutes
3x Power snatch (135#)
6x Box jumps (24 inch)
Sprint 40m

AMRAP WOD #101

Max rounds in 20 minutes
10x Burpees
15x Box jump overs (24"/20")
5x Hang squat clean (185#/125#)

AMRAP WOD #102 - Cindy's ugly cousin

Max rounds in 21 minutes
7x Pull-ups
14x Push-ups

21x Double-unders

AMRAP WOD #103
Max rounds in 25 minutes
8x Handstand push-ups
8x Box jump (30")
15 ft rope climb, 1 ascent

AMRAP WOD #104
Max rounds in 30 minutes
10x Handstand push-ups
10x Ring dips
10x Pull-ups
10x Sit-ups
10x Overhead squat (45#)
10x Double unders

AMRAP WOD #105
Max rounds in 30 minutes
Run 800m
25x Thrusters (35# DBs)
400m DB farmers carry

AMRAP WOD #106 – Hortman
Max rounds in 45 minutes
Run 800m
80x Squats
8x Muscle-ups

AMRAP WOD #107
Max rounds, no time limit
Perform one set every minute on the minute, add 10# per round until failure
2x Back squat (starting weight is 135#/85#)

AMRAP WOD #108
On the minute for max rounds
3x Back squat (75% 1RM)
40 yd sprint
5x Pull-ups, strict

AMRAP WOD #109
For max rounds
Max rounds in 4 minutes of 5x Hang squat snatch (135#/85#) + 10x Burpees
Rest 2 minutes
Max rounds in 4 minutes of 10x Power clean (135#/85#) + 20x Pull-ups
Rest 2 minutes
Max rounds in 4 minutes of 15x Box jump-overs (24/20") + 30x Wall ball (20#/14#)

AMRAP WOD #110
Max rounds, no time limit
Do one triplet every 30 seconds until failure
1x Deadlift (3/4 bw)
1x Hang clean
1x Push jerk

AMRAP WOD #111
Max rounds
5x Thruster (95#)
10x Hang power clean
15x Sumo deadlift high pull

AMRAP WOD #112
Max rounds
Rest 1 minute between rounds, add 10# per round, continue

until failure
2x Overhead squat (starting weight is 75#/45#)

Triple Element WODs

Triple Element WOD #1
5 rounds
22x Inverted burpees
22x Pull-ups
22x Sit-ups

Triple Element WOD #2
Max rounds in 20 minutes
10x Strict handstand push-ups
20x Strict pull-ups
200m Run

Triple Element WOD #3
4 rounds
Sprint 50m
4x Muscle-ups
35x Sit-ups

Triple Element WOD #4
5 rounds
50x Squats
30x Pull-ups
15x Handstand push-ups

Triple Element WOD #5
5 rounds
10x Strict pull-ups
30x Squats

30 cal row

Triple Element WOD #6
3 rounds
60-30-15x Push-ups
40-20-10 Pull-ups
20-10-5x Box jump

Triple Element WOD #7
Max rounds in 20 minutes
15x Pull-ups
30x Push-ups
25x box jumps

Triple Element WOD #8
Max rounds in 12 minutes
45x Double-unders
30x Pull-ups
15x Handstand push-ups

Triple Element WOD #9
3 rounds
21-15-9x reps
Burpee tuck-jumps

Triple Element WOD #10
Max rounds in 15 minutes
10x Muscle-ups
10x Pistol squats
50x Double-unders

Triple Element WOD #11
3 rounds
21-15-9x reps, start and finish wod with 800m run

Handstand push-ups
Burpees
Knees to elbows

Triple Element WOD #12
3 rounds
100x Squats
20x Handstand push-ups
400m Run

Triple Element WOD #13
5 rounds
21-18-15-12-9x
Knees to elbows
Ring push-ups
40 cal row

Triple Element WOD #14
7 rounds, 21-18-15-12-9-6-3x reps
Squats
Knees to elbows
Push-ups

Triple Element WOD #15
3 rounds
21-15-9x
Body-blasters (burpee + pull-up + knees to elbows)

Triple Element WOD #16
7 rounds
35x Squats
25x Push-ups
15x Pull-ups

Triple Element WOD #17
5 rounds
15x L pull-ups
30x Push-ups
45x Sit-ups

Triple Element WOD #18
Max rounds in 15 minutes
10x Muscle-ups
10x Pistol squats
10x Sit-ups

Triple Element WOD #19
For time
25x Handstand push-ups
50x Pistols, alternating
75x Pull-ups

Triple Element WOD #20
Max rounds in 20 minutes
25x Pull-ups
50x Push-ups
75x Squats

Triple Element WD #21
3 RFT
25x Box Jumps
30x Thrusters
25x Push-ups

Triple Element WD #22
3 RFT
25x Box Jumps
30x Deadlift

25x Push-ups

Triple Element WD #23
3 RFT
25x Box Jumps
30x Push press
25x Push-ups

Triple Element WD #24
3 RFT
25x Box Jumps
30x OH press
25x Push-ups

Triple Element WD #22
3 RFT
25x Box Jumps
30x OH Squat
25x Push-ups

Triple Element WD #23
3 RFT
25x Box Jumps
30x Back Extensions
25x Pull-ups

Triple Element WD #24
3 RFT
25x Box Jumps
30x Dips
25x Push-ups

Triple Element WD #25
3 RFT

25x Box Jumps
30x Wall Balls
25x Push-ups

Triple Element WD #26
3 RFT
25x Box Jumps
30x TTB
25x Push-ups

Triple Element WD #27
5 RFT
25x Double-unders
30x Thrusters
25x Air squats

Triple Element WD #28
5 RFT
25x Double-unders
30x Deadlifts
25x Air squats

Triple Element WD #29
5 RFT
25x Double-unders
30x Push press
25x Air squats

Triple Element WD #30
5 RFT
25x Double-unders
30x OH Press
25x Air squats

Triple Element WD #31
5 RFT
25x Double-unders
30x Back extensions
25x Air squats

Triple Element WD #32
5 RFT
25x Double-unders
30x Snatches
25x Air squats

Triple Element WD #33
4 RFT
25x Double-unders
30x Wall Balls
25x TTB

Triple Element WD #34
4 RFT
25x Double-unders
30x Wall Balls
25x KTE

Triple Element WD #35
5 RFT
25x Double-unders
30x Thrusters
25x Air squats

Triple Element WD #36
Max rounds in 15 minutes
30x Walking lunges with KB
30x Thrusters

25x GHD Sit-ups

Triple Element WD #37
Max rounds in 15 minutes
30x Walking lunges with KB
30x Snatches
15x Turkish get-ups

Triple Element WD #38
Max rounds in 12 minutes
30x Walking lunges with KB
30x Dips
Run 200m

Triple Element WD #39
Max rounds in 15 minutes
30x Walking lunges with KB
30x OH Squats
15x TTB

Triple Element WD #40
5 RFT
Run 400m
30x Ring rows
25x Wall balls

Triple Element WD #41
Max rounds in 15 minutes
30x Wall balls
30x Push press
50 Single-unders

Triple Element WD #42
Max rounds in 15 minutes

30x Walking lunges with KB
30x Thrusters
25x GHD Sit-ups

Triple Element WD #43
5 RFT
25 Cal row
16x C2B Pull-ups
9x HSPU

Triple Element WD #44
4 RFT
400m Run
4x Muscle-ups
40 Double-unders

Triple Element WD #45
For time
10-9-8-7-6-5-4-3-2-1
Strict Press 95/65
20-18-16-14-12-10-8-6-4-2
Ab mat sit-ups
Run 200m

Triple Element WD #46
5 RFT
3 Muscle Ups
10 Front Squats (155/105)
15 HSPU

Triple Element WD #47
7 RFT
20x Wall balls
20x Burpees

20x Ring rows

Triple Element WD #48
Max rounds in 15 minutes
15x Bar facing burpees
25x OH squats
30x Ab mat sit-ups

Triple Element WD #49
5 RFT
10 Power Snatches
15 Cal Row
20 OH Walking Lunges

Triple Element WD #50
5 RFT
400m run
21 KBS 53/35
15 Wall-balls
9 Medicine ball sit-ups

Triple Element WD #51
4 RFT
10x Power cleans
20x TTB
30x Jumping jacks

Triple Element WD #52
5 RFT
50x Single-unders
3x Rope climb
30x Wall balls

Triple Element WD #53

Max rounds in 15 minutes
75x Single-unders
25x Deadlifts
15x Burpees

Triple Element WD #54
4 RFT
100x Single-unders
20x Thrusters
20x C2B Pull-ups

Triple Element WD #55
7 RFT
75x Single-unders
20x OH Squat
20x Ring rows

Triple Element WD #56
Max rounds in 10 minutes
21x Deadlift
400m Farmers carry with KB)
15x Deadlift

Triple Element WD #57
Mac rounds in 12 minutes
1x Bar muscle-up
2x Handstand push-ups
3x Pistols

Triple Element WD #58
10 RFT
10x Pull-ups
20x Burpees
30x Sit-ups

40x Air squats

Triple Element WD #59
5 RFT
Run 200m
10x C2B Pull-ups
Run 200m
5x Power snatch (135#/95#)

Triple Element WD #60
7 RFT
40x Push-ups
50x Squats
10x Inverted burpees

Triple Element WD #61
4 RFT
Run 400m
25x Ring rows
25x Push-ups
25x GHD sit-ups
25x Squat jumps

Triple Element WD #62
Max reps in 15 minutes
10x Sumo deadlift high pull (95/65#)
10x Wall-ball (20#/14#)
20x Push-press (35#/25# DBs)

Triple Element WD #63
Max rounds in 12 minutes
2x Rope climbs
20x Walking lunge steps
Row 200m

Triple Element WD #64
3 RFT
5x Power clean (135#/95#)
10x KB swings (53#/36#)
15x Wall-ball (20#/14#)

Triple Element WD #65
3 RFT
50x Double-unders
30x Hand-release push-ups
20x Ring dips

Triple Element WD #66
Max rounds in 10 minutes
3x Power clean (60% 1RM)
5x Pull-ups
10x Burpees

Tabata WODs

Tabata WOD #1
For max distance
Row 8x [20:10]

Tabata WOD #2
For max reps
8x [20:10]* Deadlifts (315#+)

Tabata WOD #3
For max reps/cals
Double KB thrusters (36#/24#) 8x [20:10]
Rest 3 minutes

Row or Airdyne 8x [20:10]
Rest 4 minutes
Double-unders 8x [20:10]

Tabata WOD #4
For max reps
Pull-ups 8x [20:10]
Rest 3 minutes
Squats 8x [20:10]
Rest 3 minutes
Push-ups 8x [20:10]

Tabata WOD #5
For max reps/cals
Double unders 8x [20:10]
Rest 2 minutes
Squats 8x [20:10]
Rest 2 minutes
Row 8x [20:10]

Tabata WOD #6
For max reps
Back squat (135#/95) 8x [20:10]
Bar must stay on back throughout entire WOD

Tabata WOD #7
For max reps
Pull-ups 8x [20:10]
Rest 3 minutes
Squats 8x [20:10]
Rest 3 minutes
Push-ups 8x [20:10]

Tabata WOD #8

For max reps
KB snatch (36#/24#) 8x [20:10]
Switch hands each interval

Tabata WOD #9
2 rounds
4x [20:10] Row, AirDyne, or Assault bike for calories
Rest 1 minute
4x [20:10] Max reps GHD sit-ups
Rest 1 minute
4x [20:10] Max reps Double unders
Rest 1 minute
4x [20:10] Max reps wall ball (20#/14#)
Rest 2 minutes

Tabata WOD #10 - Tabata up Yours
For max reps
Deadlift (135#/95#) 8x [20:10]
Rest 4 minutes
Push press (75#/55#) 8x [20:10]
Rest 4 minutes
Box jumps (20/16 inch) 8x [20:10]
Rest 4 minutes
Ball slam (30#/20#) 8x [20:10]

Tabata WOD #11 - Tabata Fight Gone Bad
Wall balls (20#/14#) 8x [20:10]
SDHP (75# / 55#) 8x [20:10]
Box Jumps (20 / 16) 8x [20:10]
Push Presses (75# / 55#) 8x [20:10
Row 8x [20:10]

Tabata WOD #12
Back Squats (135# / 95#) 8x [20:10]

Shoulder-to-overheads (135# / 95#) 8x [20:10]
Rest with bar in the rack position (front rack for should-to-OH and back rack for back squats)

Tabata WOD #13
Thrusters (45# / 35#) 8x [20:10]
Pull-ups 8x [20:10]
Thrusters (45# / 35#) 8x [20:10]
Push-ups 8x [20:10]

Tabata WOD #14
Ball Slams (30# / 20#) 8x [20:10]
Wall Ball Shots (20# / 14#) 8x [20:10]

Advanced WODs

Advanced WODs are the most difficult to complete. These are the workouts that only seasoned athletes will be doing. The weights are heavier and there are more reps. The times are longer and more equipment is needed. Also, the moves are more technical. It is important with these workouts to have good form going into this level of work, because bad form at such high intensity can result in poor performance at least and potential injury at worst. Remember the importance of your preparations with these workouts, as you will be challenging your body significantly and you need to have the muscles prepared to perform the advanced movements that you are going to be asking it to do.

Olympic Lifting WODs

Olympic WOD #1
15 min to work to 1RM
Snatch

Olympic WOD #2
15 in to work to 3RM
Snatch

Olympic WOD #3
For time
15x Snatch

Olympic WOD #4
12 min to work to heavy single
Hang Snatch

Olympic WOD #5
12 min to work 3RM

Hang Snatch

Olympic WOD #6
10 min to work to 1RM
Clean

Olympic WOD #7
12 min to work to 3RM
Clean

Olympic WOD #8
For time
30x Clean

Olympic WOD #9
15 minutes to work to 1RM
Clean and Jerk

Olympic WOD #10
20 minutes to work to 3RM
Clean and Jerk

Olympic WOD #11
For time
50x Clean and Jerks

Olympic WOD #12
12 minutes to work to
3 position Clean and 1 Jerk

Olympic WOD #13
12 minutes to work 3RD
Hang Clean and Jerk

Olympic WOD #14 - Spinning Grace
For time
30x Clean & jerk (135#)
After each lockout you must rotate 360-degrees with bar in overhead position

Olympic WOD #15
7 rounds for max reps
1 minute max reps squat clean starting at 135#/85#
Rest 3 minutes
Continue up ladder adding 20# to the bar each round thereafter
7 rounds total, last round will be 255#/205#

Olympic WOD #16
Rest as needed between lifts
Clean & jerk 1-1-1-1-1x reps

Olympic WOD #17 - Bob's Tasty Combo #11
Rest as needed between efforts
Power snatch 3-3-3-3-3x @ 65% 1RM
Jerk 3-3-3-3-3x @ 60% 1RM
Clean high pull from floor 4-4-4-4-4x @ 90% 1RM
Back squat 8-8-8-6-6x @ 60% 1RM

Olympic WOD #18 - Bob's Tasty Combo #12
Rest as needed between efforts
Power snatch + overhead squat 3-3-3-3-3x @ 65% snatch 1RM
Jerk 2-2-2-2x @ 70% 1RM
DB windmill 5-5-5x per side @ 40#

Olympic WOD #19
For max reps
10 minute time cap

30x Snatch (75#/45#)
30x Snatch (135#/75#)
30x Snatch (165#/100#)
Max reps Snatch (210#/120#)

Olympic WOD #20 - Bob's Tasty Combo #6
Rest as needed between efforts
Snatch 2x @ 70% 1RM, 2x @ 75%, 2x @ 77%
Clean & jerk 2x @ 70% 1RM, 2x @ 75%, 2x @ 77%

Olympic WOD #21 - Bob's Tasty Combo #3
Rest as needed between efforts
Snatch 3-3-3x @ 70% 1RM
Snatch high pull of blocks 3-3-3x @ 80% 1RM
Snatch push jerk, behind neck 4-4-4-4x @ 50% 1RM

Olympic WOD #22
Work up to a max load, rest exactly 2 minutes between lifts
Snatch grip deadlift 1RM

Olympic WOD #23 - Bob's Tasty Combo #2
Heavy singles, rest as needed between efforts
Snatch 1-1-1-1-1x
Clean & jerk 1-1-1-1-1x
Back squat 1-1-1-1-1x

Olympic WOD #24 - Bob's Tasty Combo #8
Rest as needed between efforts
Snatch 1-1-1-1-1x @ 80% 1RM
Snatch high pull off blocks 3-3-3x @ 90% 1RM
Back squat 2-2-2-2x @ 87% 1RM

Olympic WOD #25
2 rounds

1 minute max reps squat clean (165#)
Rest 3 minutes
1 minute max reps squat clean (185#)
Rest 3 minutes
1 minute max reps squat clean (205#)
Rest 3 minutes

Olympic WOD #26
7 rounds for max reps
1 minute max reps squat clean starting at 135#/85#
Rest 3 minutes
Continue up ladder adding 20# to the bar each round thereafter
7 rounds total, last round will be 255#/205#

Olympic WOD #27
5 rounds
Rest as needed between lifts
Clean & jerk 1-1-1-1-1x reps

Olympic WOD #28 - Bob's Tasty Combo #1
Rest as needed between efforts
Snatch 2-2-2-2x @ 75% 1RM
Jerk 2-2-2-2-2x @ 80% 1RM
Clean high pull from blocks 3-3-3x @ 90% 1RM
Back squat 2-2-2-2x @ 90% 1RM

Olympic WOD #29
For time
30x Curtis Press (95#)
(1x Curtis Press = 1x hang power clean + 1x right leg lunge + 1x left leg lunge + 1x push-press)

Olympic WOD #30 - Double Grace

For time
60x Clean & jerks (135#/95#)

Strongman WODs

Strongman WOD #1
8 rounds
50-ft' Zercher yoke carry (as heavy as possible)
12x Ring dips

Strongman WOD #2
9 rounds
50 ft Zercher yoke carry (2x bw or higher)
3x Atlas stone ground to shoulder (bw)
Rest 1 minute

Strongman WOD #3
8 rounds
3x Axle deadlift (as heavy as possible)
100 ft Sandbag carry (bw)

Strongman WOD #4
5 rounds
10-8-6-4-2x Log viper press (150#)
50 ft Sled push (2x bw)

Strongman WOD #5
For max reps
Tabata Atlas stone ground to shoulder (145#/95#)

Strongman WOD #6
For time
Row 750m

100m Zercher yoke carry
Row 750m

Strongman WOD #7
5 rounds
1-2-3-4-5x Tire flip (3x bw)
5-4-3-2-1x Atlas stone ground to shoulder (bw)

Strongman WOD #8 - Farmers Walk Ladder
For time
300 ft Farmers walk (70#/hand)
200 ft Farmers walk (100#/hand)
100 ft Farmers walk (200#/hand)
50 ft Farmers walk (250#/hand)
For each drop do 5x burpee penalty on the spot.

Strongman WOD #9
For max reps
Tabata Axle deadlift (300#)

Strongman WOD #10
EMOM for 20 minutes
1x Back squat (405#)
1x Stone ground to shoulder (AHAP)

Strongman WOD #11
6 rounds
5x Bench Press (275#)
10x KB Swings (106#)
50 ft Duck walk (250#)

Strongman WOD #12
3 rounds
5x Tire flip (2x bw)

15x Burpees
4x Tire flip (3x bw)
10x Burpees
3x Tire flip (4x bw)
5x Burpees
Rest 2 minutes between rounds

Strongman WOD #13
EMOM for 12 minutes
75 ft Farmers walk (250# per hand)
After completion rest 5 minutes then repeat with 75 ft yoke carry (3x bw)

Strongman WOD #14
12 minutes AMRAP
100 ft Farmers walk (100#/hand)
12x KB swings (106#)

Strongman WOD #15
3 rounds
Keg over 45 inch bar (AHAP)
Row 30 cals
40x KB swings (53#)
50x Push-ups

Strongman WOD #16
3 rounds
50 ft Farmers walk (2x bw per hand)
10x GHD sit-ups
Rest 2 minutes

Strongman WOD #17
5 rounds
6x/shoulder Single-sided Atlas stone squat (175# or higher)

12x GHD sit-ups

Strongman WOD #18
6 rounds
10x Bench press
10x Chest to bar pull-ups
100 ft odd object carry (bw)

Strongman WOD #19
3 rounds
Max duration overhead axle hold (bw)
Rest 3 minutes
Max duration static crucifix hold (25# per hand)
Rest 3 minutes

Strongman WOD #20
5 rounds
3x Sumo deadlift (415#/275#)
5x Stone ground to shoulder (AHAP)
60 ft Yoke carry, anyhow (AHAP)
Rest 2 minutes

Strongman WOD #21
For time
800m Sandbag carry (50% bw)
400m Atlas stone carry (75% bw)
200m Sled push (2x bw)
Rest 60 sec between implements, subtract rest from total time.

Strongman WOD #22
4 rounds
100 ft Zercher carry (AHAP)
Row 250m
Rest 60 seconds

Strongman WOD #23
5 rounds
5x Log clean and press (80% 1RM)
50 ft Duck walk (250#)

Strongman WOD #24
5 rounds
5x Thrusters (bw)
5x Axle deadlifts (2x bw)
Scale up or down as needed.

Strongman WOD #25
4 rounds
12-9-6-3x reps
Tire flips (3x bw)
Front Squat @ 1.25X BWT (or more)
Bar muscle ups

Strongman WOD #26 - Tatts
5 rounds
250-200-150-100-50 ft Yoke carry (300-400-500-600-700#)
10-8-6-4-2x Back squat (225-275-315-365-405#)

Strongman WOD #27 - 3000
For time
Using a yoke move 3000# of weight 75 ft
Start by stacking 3000# worth of plates at a starting line.
Start a clock then load the yoke with whatever you can carry and move it 75 ft.
Empty the yoke, carry it back, reload, and continue until all weight is moved.

Strongman WOD #28

For time
50x Axle front squats (225#)
50x Weighted dips (90#)
Row 50 calories

Strongman WOD #29
For time
400m Atlas stone carry (bw)

Strongman WOD #30
EMOM for 30 minutes
First minute - 3x Log ground to overhead (bw)
Second minute - 3x Front squats (1.25x bw)
Third minute - 8x Strict pull-ups

Strongman WOD #31
5 rounds
100 ft Keg carry (5x burpees per drop)
5x/arm DB snatch (80#)
Rest 60 seconds

Strongman WOD #32
6 rounds
3x Axle power clean (185#/115#)
4x Elevated knee jumps
50 ft Odd object carry (bw)

Strongman WOD #33
4 rounds
100 ft Backward sled drag (AHAP)
3x Axle deadlift (2x bw)
100 ft Forward sled push
3 Axle deadlift
Rest 2 minutes

Strongman WOD #34
For time
15x Tire flips (3x bw)
Row 1000m
15x Tire flips (3x bw)

Strongman WOD #35 – Jake
7 rounds
3x Muscle-ups
2x Tire flips (3x bw)
1x Atlas stone ground to shoulder (bw)

Powerlifting WODs

Powerlifting WOD #1
For time
52x Squats (135#)

Powerlifting WOD #2
For time
100x Thruster (95#)

Powerlifting WOD #3
7 x 5 @ 75% of 1RM
+ 5 Box Jumps after each set.
Rear Foot Elevated Split Squat

Powerlifting WOD #4
Bench Press - 12 x 2 @ 50%

Powerlifting WOD #5
Deadlift - 5 x 3 @ 85% of 1RM

+ 5 Broad Jump after each set.

Powerlifting WOD #6
Overhead Press - 5 x 5 @ 75%
5 x 5 Kipping Handstand Push Ups @ Max Depth

Powerlifting WOD #7
Front Squat - 4 x 12 (Use Chart)
12 Overhead Lunge after each set

Powerlifting WOD #8
Back Squat - 4 x 12 (use the chart)
*Super set each set with 20 Overhead Squat with a Pipe

Powerlifting WOD #9
Bench Press - 6 x 6 @ 70%
*Super set each set with a 50m overhead carry.

Powerlifting WOD #10
Deadlift - 15 x 2 @ 50%
Reps are done for speed. 20 second rest between sets.

Powerlifting WOD #11
Front Squat - 3 x 2 @ 90%

Powerlifting WOD #12
Back Squat - 3 sets of 5 reps @ 85% of 1RM
*Super Set with 5 Box Jumps
Rear Foot Elevated Split Squat
3 x 10 Each Leg

Powerlifting WOD #13
Bench Press - 5 sets of 3 reps @ 85% of 1RM
*Super set with 5 Plyo Push Ups

Powerlifting WOD #14
Barbell Row - 5 sets of 5 reps

Powerlifting WOD #15
Deadlift - 6 sets of 6 reps @ 70% of 1RM
*Super Set with 5 max effort broad jumps

Powerlifting WOD #16
Overhead Press - 4 sets of 12 reps
3 Max Handstand Holds

Powelifting WOD #17
Front Squat - 5 sets of 5 reps @ 70% of 1RM
*2 second pause in the hold of each rep
Rear Foot Elevated Split Squat
5 sets of 5 reps each leg

Powerlifting WOD #18
Bench Press - 5 x 5 @ 80% of 1RM
**Do 1 set every 90 seconds

Powerlifting WOD #19
Back Squat - 5 x 3 @ 85% + 5 Plyos

Powerlifting WOD #20
EMOM for 20 minutes
3 Back Squat @ 50%
2 Snatch High Pull + 2 Snatch + 2 Overhead Squat @ 60%

Heros WODs

Hero WOD #1 – Omar

3 rounds
Thruster (95#) 10-20-30x
Bar-facing burpees 15-25-35x

Hero WOD #2 – Nick
12 rounds
10x Hang squat clean (45# DBs)
6x Handstand push-ups on the DBS

Hero WOD #3 – Ozzy
7 rounds
11x Deficit handstand push-ups
Run 1km

Hero WOD #4 – RJ
5 rounds
Run 800m
15 ft rope climb, 5 ascents
50x Push-ups

Hero WOD #5 – Bruck
4 rounds
Run 400m
24x Back squat (185#)
24x Jerk (135#)

Hero WOD #6 – Luce
3 rounds
Wear 20# vest
Run 1K
10x Muscle-ups
100x Squats

Hero WOD #7 – Garrett

3 rounds
75x Squats
25x Ring handstand push-ups
25x L pull-ups

Hero WOD #8 – Roy
5 rounds
15x Deadlift (225#)
20x Box jumps (24 inch)
25x Pull-ups

Hero WOD #9 – Luke
For time
Run 400m
15x Clean & jerk (155#)
Run 400m
30x Toes to bar
Run 400m
45x Wall ball (20#)
Run 400m
45x KB swings (53#)
Run 400m
30x Ring dips
Run 400m
15x Walking lunges (155#)
Run 400m

Hero WOD #10 – McGhee
Max rounds in 30 minutes
5x Deadlifts (275#)
13x Push-ups
9x Box jumps (24 inch)

Hero WOD #11 – Hansen

5 rounds
30x KB swing (72#)
30x Burpees
30x GHD sit-ups

Hero WOD #12 - Adam Brown
2 rounds
7x Deadlift (295#)
7x Box jumps (24 inch)
7x Wall ball (20#)
7x Bench press (195#)
7x Box jumps
7x Wall ball
7x Clean (145#)

Hero WOD #13 – Loredo
6 rounds
24x Squats
24x Push-ups
24x Walking lunge steps
Run 400m

Hero WOD #14 – Sean
10 rounds
11x chest-to-bar pull-ups
22x Front squat (75#)

Hero WOD #15 – Santora
3 rounds
1 minute each for max reps
Squat cleans (155#)
20 ft Shuttle sprints (20 ft forward + 20 ft backwards = 1 rep)
Jerk (155#)
Rest 1 minute

Hero WOD #16 – Johnson

Max rounds in 20 minutes
9x Deadlift (245#)
8x Muscle-ups
9x Squat clean (155#)

Hero WOD #17 – Jbo

Max rounds in 28 minutes
9x Overhead squat (115#)
15 ft legless rope climb, 1 ascent
12x Bench press (115#)

Hero WOD #18 – Daniel

For time
50x Pull-ups
21x Thruster (95#)
Run 800m
21x Thruster
Run 400m
50x Pull-ups

Hero WOD #19 – Zimmerman

Max rounds in 25 minutes
11x Chest-to-bar pull-ups
2x Deadlift (315#)
10x Handstand push-ups

Hero WOD #20 – Bradley

10 rounds
Sprint 100m
10x Pull-ups
Sprint 100m
10x Burpees

Rest 30 seconds

Hero WOD #21 – Coffey
3 rounds
Run 800 meters
50-35-20x Back squat (135#)
50-35-20x Bench press (135#)

Finish triplet with an additional 800m run and 1x Muscle-up

Hero WOD #22 – Severin
For time
Wear body armor or 20# vest if available.
50x Strict pull-ups
100x Push-ups, release hands from floor at bottom
Run 5K

Hero WOD #23 – White
5 rounds
15 foot Rope climb, 3 ascents
10x Toes to bar
21x Overhead walking lunges (45# plate)
Run 400m

Hero WOD #24 – Weston
5 rounds
Row 1000m
200m Farmers walk (2x45# DBs)
50m Waiter walk, right arm (45# DB)
50m Waiter walk, right arm (45# DB)

Hero WOD #25 – Shawn
For time
Run 5 miles

Stop every 5 minutes and do 50x squats and 50x push-ups

Hero WOD #26 – Falkel
Max rounds in 25 minutes
8x Handstand push-ups
8x Box jump (30")
15 ft rope climb, 1 ascent

Hero WOD #27 – Jason
4 rounds
Squats 100-75-50-25x reps
Muscle-ups 5-10-15-20x reps

Hero WOD #28 – Strange
8 rounds
Run 600m
11x Weighted pull-ups (53# KB)
11x Walking lunges (2x53#KBs)
11x KB Thruster (2x53#)

Hero WOD #29 - Lumberjack 20
5 rounds
20x Deadlifts (275#)
Run 400m
20x KB swings (72#)
Run 400m
Overhead squat (115#)
Run 400m
20x Burpees
Run 400m
20x Pull-ups
Run 400m
20x Box jumps (24 inch)
Run 400m

20x DB squat cleans (45# DBs)
Run 400m

Hero WOD #30 – Tyler
5 rounds
7x Muscle-ups
21x Sumo deadlift high-pull (95#)

Hero WOD #31 – Capoot
4 rounds
100-75-50-25x Push-ups
Run 800-1200-1600-2000m

Hero WOD #32 – Wyk
5 rounds
5x Front squat (225#), 5x 15-ft Rope climb, Run 400m with a 45# plate

Hero WOD #33 – Spehar
For time
100x Thruster (135#)
100x Chest to bar pull-ups
Run 6 miles

Hero WOD #34 – JT
21-15-9 reps, for time
Handstand push-ups
Ring dips
Push-ups

Hero WOD #35
3 RFT
Run 800 meters
50 Back Extensions

50 Sit-ups

Hero WOD #36 – Murph
For time
Partition the pull-ups, push-ups, and squats as needed. Start and finish with a mile run. If you've got a twenty pound vest or body armor, wear it.
1 mile Run
100 Pull-ups
200 Push-ups
300 Squats
1 mile Run

Hero WOD #37 – Josh
For time
95 pound Overhead squat, 21 reps
42 Pull-ups
95 pound Overhead squat, 15 reps
30 Pull-ups
95 pound Overhead squat, 9 reps
18 Pull-ups

Hero WOD #38 - Badger
3RFT
95 pound Squat clean, 30 reps
30 Pull-ups
Run 800 meters

Hero WOD #39 – Joshie
3RFT
40 pound Dumbbell snatch, 21 reps, right arm
21 L Pull-ups
40 pound Dumbbell snatch, 21 reps, left arm
21 L Pull-ups

The snatches are full squat snatches.

Hero WOD #40 – Nate
20 Minute AMRAP
2 Muscle-ups
4 Handstand Push-ups
8 2-Pood Kettlebell swings

Hero WOD #41 – Randy
For time
75# power snatch, 75 reps

Hero WOD #42 – Tommy V
For time
115 pound Thruster, 21 reps
15 ft Rope Climb, 12 ascents
115 pound Thruster, 15 reps
15 ft Rope Climb, 9 ascents
115 pound Thruster, 9 reps
15 ft Rope Climb, 6 ascents

Hero WOD #43 – Griff
For time
Run 800 meters
Run 400 meters backwards
Run 800 meters
Run 400 meters backwards

Hero WOD #44 - Ryan
7 Muscle-ups
21 Burpees
Each burpee terminates with a jump one foot above max standing reach.

Hero WOD #45 – Erin
5 RFT
40 pound Dumbbells split clean, 15 reps
21 Pull-ups

Hero WOD #46 – Mr. Joshua
5 RFT
Run 400 meters
30 Glute-ham sit-ups
250 pound Deadlift, 15 reps

Hero WOD #47 – DT
5 RFT
155 pound Deadlift, 12 reps
155 pound Hang power clean, 9 reps
155 pound Push jerk, 6 reps

Hero WOD #48 – Danny
20 minute AMRAP
24" box jump, 30 reps
115 pound push press, 20 reps
30 pull-ups

Hero WOD #49 – Hansen
5 RFT
30 reps, 2 pood Kettlebell swing
30 Burpees
30 Glute-ham sit-ups

Hero WOD #50 – Stephen
For time
30-25-20-15-10-5 rep rounds of:
GHD sit-up

Back extension
Knees to elbow
95 pound Stiff legged deadlift

Hero WOD #51 – War Frank
3 RFT
25 Muscle-ups
100 Squats
35 GHD situps

Hero WOD #52 – Paul
5 RFT
50 Double unders
35 Knees to elbows
185 pound Overhead walk, 20 yards

Hero WOD #53 – Jerry
For time
Run 1 mile
Row 2K
Run 1 mile

Hero WOD #54 – Nutts
For time
10 Handstand push-ups
250 pound Deadlift, 15 reps
25 Box jumps, 30 inch box
50 Pull-ups
100 Wallball shots, 20 pounds, 10'
200 Double-unders
Run 400 meters with a 45lb plate

Hero WOD #55 – Arnie
For time

With a single 2 pood kettlebell:
21 Turkish get-ups, Right arm
50 Swings
21 Overhead squats, Left arm
50 Swings
21 Overhead squats, Right arm
50 Swings
21 Turkish get-ups, Left arm

Hero WOD #56 – The Seven
7 RFT
7 Handstand push-ups
135 pound Thruster, 7 reps
7 Knees to elbows
245 pound Deadlift, 7 reps
7 Burpees
7 Kettlebell swings, 2 pood
7 Pull-ups

Hero WOD #57 – Roy
5 RFT
225 pound Deadlift, 15 reps
20 Box jumps, 24 inch box
25 Pull-ups

Hero WOD #58 – Coe
10 RFT
95 pound Thruster, 10 reps
10 Ring push-ups

Hero WOD #59 – Helton
3 RFT
Run 800 meters
30 reps, 50 pound dumbbell squat cleans

30 Burpees

Hero WOD #60 – Jack
20 minute AMRAP
115 pound Push press, 10 reps
10 KB Swings, 1.5 pood
10 Box jumps, 24 inch box
Forrest
3 RFT
20 L-pull-ups
30 Toes to bar
40 Burpees
Run 800 meters

Hero WOD #61 – Bulger
10 RFT
Run 150 meters
7 Chest to bar pull-ups
135 pound Front squat, 7 reps
7 Handstand push-ups

Hero WOD #62 – Brenton
5 RFT
Run 150 meters
7 Chest to bar pull-ups
135 pound Front squat, 7 reps
7 Handstand push-ups

Hero WOD #63 – Blake
4 RFT
100 foot Walking lunge with 45lb plate held overhead
30 Box jump, 24 inch box
20 Wallball shots, 20 pound ball
10 Handstand push-ups

Hero WOD #64 – Collin
6 RFT
Carry 50 pound sandbag 400 meters
115 pound Push press, 12 reps
12 Box jumps, 24 inch box
95 pound Sumo deadlift high-pull, 12 reps

Hero WOD #65 – Thompson
10 RFT
95 pound Back squat, 29 reps
135 pound barbells Farmer carry, 10 meters
Begin the rope climbs seated on the floor.

Hero WOD #66 – Blake Whitten
5 RFT
22 Kettlebell swings, 2 pood
22 Box jump, 24 inch box
Run 400 meters
22 Burpees
22 Wall ball shots, 20 pound ball

Hero WOD #67 – Bull
2 RFT
135 pound Overhead squat, 50 reps
50 Pull-ups
Run 1 mile

Hero WOD #68 – Rankel
20 minute AMRAP
225 pound Deadlift, 6 reps
7 Burpee pull-ups
10 Kettlebell swings, 2 pood
Run 200 meters

Hero WOD #69 – Holbrook
10 RFT, each round for time
115 pound Thruster, 5 reps
10 Pull-ups
100 meter Sprint
Rest 1 minute

Hero WOD #70 – Ledesma
20 minute AMRAP
5 Parallette handstand push-ups
10 Toes through rings
20 pound Medicine ball cleans, 15 reps

Hero WOD #71 – Whittman
7 RFT
1.5 pood Kettlebell swing, 15 reps
95 pound Power clean, 15 reps
15 Box jumps, 24″ box

Hero WOD #72 – McCluskey
3 RFT
9 Muscle-ups
15 Burpee pull-ups
21 Pull-ups
Run 800 meters

Hero WOD #73 – Weaver
4 RFT
10 L-pull-ups
15 Push-ups
15 Chest to bar Pull-ups
15 Push-ups
20 Pull-ups

15 Push-ups

Hero WOD #74 – Abbate
For time
Run 1 mile
155 pound Clean and jerk, 21 reps
Run 800 meters
155 pound Clean and jerk, 21 reps
Run 1 Mile

Hero WOD #75 – Hammer
5 RFT, each round for time
135 pound Power clean, 5 reps
135 pound Front squat, 10 reps
135 pound Jerk, 5 reps
20 Pull-ups
Rest 90 seconds between each round

Hero WOD #76 – Moore
20 minute AMRAP
15 ft Rope Climb, 1 ascent
Run 400 meters
Max rep Handstand push-ups

Hero WOD #77 – Wilmot
6 RFT
25 Ring dips

Hero WOD #78 – Moon
7 RFT
15 ft Rope Climb, 1 ascent
40 pound dumbbell Hang split snatch, 10 reps Left arm
15 ft Rope Climb, 1 ascent
Alternate feet in the split snatch sets.

Hero WOD #79 – Small
3 RFT
Row 1000 meters
50 Burpees
50 Box jumps, 24" box
Run 800 meters

Hero WOD #80 – Morrison
For Time
50-40-30-20 and 10 rep rounds of:
Wall ball shots, 20 pound ball
Box jump, 24 inch box
Kettlebell swings, 1.5 pood

Hero WOD #81 – Manion
7 RFT
Run 400 meters
135 pound Back squat, 29 reps

Hero WOD #82 – Gator
8 RFT
185 pound Front squat, 5 reps
26 Ring push-ups

Hero WOD #83 – Meadows
For Time
20 Muscle-ups
25 Lowers from an inverted hang on the rings, slowly, with straight body and arms
30 Ring handstand push-ups
35 Ring rows
40 Ring push-ups

Hero WOD #84 – Santiago
7 RFT
35 pound Dumbbell hang squat clean, 18 reps
18 Pull-ups
135 pound Power clean, 10 reps
10 Handstand push-ups

Hero WOD #85 – Carse
For Time
21-18-15-12-9-6-3 reps of:
95 pound Squat clean
Double-under
185 pound Deadlift
24" Box jump
Begin each round with a 50 meter Bear crawl.

Hero WOD #86 – Bradshaw
10 RFT
10 rounds of:
3 Handstand push-ups
225 pound Deadlift, 6 reps
12 Pull-ups
24 Double-unders

Hero WOD #87 – Wood
5 RFT
Run 400 meters
10 Burpee box jumps, 24" box
95 pound Sumo-deadlift high-pull, 10 reps
95 pound Thruster, 10 reps
Rest 1 minute

Hero WOD #88 – Hidalgo
For Time

Run 2 miles
Rest 2 minutes
135 pound Squat clean, 20 reps
20 Box jump, 24" box
20 Walking lunge steps with 45lb plate held overhead
20 Box jump, 24" box
135 pound Squat clean, 20 reps
Rest 2 minutes
Run 2 miles
If you've got a twenty pound vest or body armor, wear it.

Hero WOD #89 – Ricky
20 minute AMRAP
10 Pull-ups
75 pound dumbbell Deadlift, 5 reps
135 pound Push-press, 8 reps

Hero WOD #90 – Dae Han
3 RFT
Run 800 meters with a 45 pound barbell
15 foot Rope climb, 3 ascents
135 pound Thruster, 12 reps

Hero WOD #91 – Deforges
5 RFT
225 pound Deadlift, 12 reps
20 Pull-ups
135 pound Clean and jerk, 12 reps
20 Knees to elbows

Hero WOD #92 – Rahoi
12 minute AMRAP
24 inch Box Jump, 12 reps
95 pound Thruster, 6 reps

6 Bar-facing burpees

Hero WOD #93 – Klepto
4 RFT
27 Box jumps, 24" box
20 Burpees
11 Squat cleans, 145 pounds

Hero WOD #94 – Del
For Time
25 Burpees
Run 400 meters with a 20 pound medicine ball
25 Weighted pull-ups with a 20 pound dumbbell
Run 400 meters with a 20 pound medicine ball
25 Handstand push-ups
Run 400 meters with a 20 pound medicine ball
25 Chest-to-bar pull-ups
Run 400 meters with a 20 pound medicine ball
25 Burpees

Hero WOD #95 – Pheezy
3 RFT
165 pound Front squat, 5 reps
18 Pull-ups
225 pound Deadlift, 5 reps
18 Toes-to-bar
165 pound Push jerk, 5 reps
18 Hand-release push-ups

Hero WOD #96 – J.J.
For Time
185 pound Squat clean, 1 rep
10 Parallette handstand push-ups
185 pound Squat clean, 2 reps

9 Parallette handstand push-ups
185 pound Squat clean, 3 reps
8 Parallette handstand push-ups
185 pound Squat clean, 4 reps
7 Parallette handstand push-ups
185 pound Squat clean, 5 reps
6 Parallette handstand push-ups
185 pound Squat clean, 6 reps
5 Parallette handstand push-ups
185 pound Squat clean, 7 reps
4 Parallette handstand push-ups
185 pound Squat clean, 8 reps
3 Parallette handstand push-ups
185 pound Squat clean, 9 reps
2 Parallette handstand push-ups
185 pound Squat clean, 10 reps
1 Parallette handstand push-up

Hero WOD #97 – Jag 28
For Time
Run 800 meters
28 Kettlebell swings, 2 pood
28 Strict Pull-ups
28 Kettlebell clean and jerk, 2 pood each
28 Strict Pull-ups
Run 800 meters

Hero WOD #98 – Brian
3 RFT
15 foot Rope climb, 5 ascents
185 pound Back squat, 25 reps

Hero WOD #99 – Tumilson
8 RFT

Run 200 meters
11 Dumbbell burpee deadlifts, 60 pound dumbbells

Hero WOD #100 – Ship
9 RFT
185 pound Squat clean, 7 reps
8 Burpee box jumps, 36″ box

Hero WOD #101 – Jared
4 RFT
Run 800 meters
40 Pull-ups
70 Push-ups

Hero WOD #102 – Tully
4 RFT
Swim 200 meters
40 pound Dumbbell squat cleans, 23 reps

Hero WOD #103 – Holleyman
30 RFT
5 Wall ball shots, 20 pound ball
3 Handstand push-ups
225 pound Power clean, 1 rep

Hero WOD #104 – Adrian
7 RFT
3 Forward rolls
5 Wall climbs
7 Toes to bar
9 Box jumps, 30″ box

Hero WOD #105 – Glen
For Time

135 pound Clean and jerk, 30 reps
Run 1 mile
15 foot Rope climb, 10 ascents
Run 1 mile
100 Burpees

Hero WOD #106 – Tom
25 minute AMRAP
7 Muscle-ups
155 pound Thruster, 11 reps
14 Toes-to-bar

Hero WOD #107 – Ralph
4 RFT
250 pound Deadlift, 8 reps
16 Burpees
15 foot Rope climb, 3 ascents
Run 600 meters

Hero WOD #108 – Clovis
For Time
Run 10 miles
150 Burpee pull-ups
Partition the run and burpee pull-ups as needed.

Hero WOD #109 – Weston
5 RFT
Row 1000 meters
200 meter Farmer carry, 45 pound dumbbells
45 pound dumbbell Waiter walk, 50 meters, Right arm
45 pound dumbbell Waiter walk, 50 meters, Left arm

Hero WOD #110 – Hortman
45 minute AMRAP

Run 800 meters
80 Squats
8 Muscle-ups

Hero WOD #111 – Hamilton
3 RFT
Row 1000 meters
50 Push-ups
Run 1000 meters
50 Pull-ups

Hero WOD #112 – Zeus
3 RFT
30 Wall ball shots, 20 pound ball
75 pound Sumo deadlift high-pull, 30 reps
30 Box jump, 20" box
75 pound Push press, 30 reps
Row 30 calories
30 Push-ups
Body weight Back squat, 10 reps

Hero WOD #113 – Barraza
18 minute AMRAP
Run 200 meters
275 pound Deadlift, 9 reps
6 Burpee bar muscle-ups

Hero WOD #114 – Cameron
For Time
50 Walking lunge steps
25 Chest to bar pull-ups
50 Box jumps, 24 inch box
25 Triple-unders
50 Back extensions

25 Ring dips
50 Knees to elbows
25 Wallball "2-fer-1s", 20 pound ball
50 Sit-ups
15 foot Rope climb, 5 ascents

Hero WOD #115 – Jorge
For Time
30 GHD sit-ups
155 pound Squat clean, 15 reps
24 GHD sit-ups
155 pound Squat clean, 12 reps
18 GHD sit-ups
155 pound Squat clean, 9 reps
12 GHD sit-ups
155 pound Squat clean, 6 reps
6 GHD sit-ups
155 pound Squat clean, 3 reps

Hero WOD #116 – Brehm
For Time
15 foot Rope climb, 10 ascents
225 pound Back squat, 20 reps
30 Handstand push-ups
Row 40 calories

Hero WOD #117 – Gallant
For Time
Run 1 mile with a 20 pound medicine ball
60 Burpee pull-ups
Run 800 meters with a 20 pound medicine ball
30 Burpee pull-ups
Run 400 meters with a 20 pound medicine ball
15 Burpee pull-ups

Hero WOD #118 – Smykowski
For Time
Run 6k
60 Burpee pull-ups

Hero WOD #119 – Donny
For Time
21-15-9-9-15-21 reps of:
225 pound Deadlift
Burpee

Hero WOD #120 – Dobogai
7 RFT
8 Muscle-ups
22 yard Farmer carry, 50 pound dumbbells

Hero WOD #121 – Roney
4 RFT
Run 200 meters
135 pound Thruster, 11 reps
Run 200 meters
135 pound Push press, 11 reps
Run 200 meters
135 pound Bench press, 11 reps

Hero WOD #122 – Don
For Time
66 Deadlifts, 110 pounds
66 Box jump, 24 inch box
66 Kettlebell swings, 1.5 pood
66 Knees to elbows
66 Sit-ups
66 Pull-ups

66 Thrusters, 55 pounds
66 Wall ball shots, 20 pound ball
66 Burpees
66 Double-unders

Hero WOD #123 – Dragon
Post Load and Time
Run 5k
4 minutes to find 4 rep max Deadlift
Run 5k
4 minutes to find 4 rep max Push jerk

Hero WOD #124 – Walsh
4 RFT
22 Burpee pull-ups
185 pound Back squat, 22 reps
Run 200 meters with a 45 pound plate overhead

Hero WOD #125 – Lee
5 RFT
Run 400 meters
345 pound Deadlift, 1 rep
185 pound Squat clean, 3 reps
185 pound Push jerk, 5 reps
3 Muscle-ups
15 foot Rope climb, 1 ascent

Hero WOD #126 – Willy
3 RFT
225 pound Front squat, 5 reps
Run 200 meters
11 Chest to bar pull-ups
Run 400 meters
12 Kettlebell swings, 2 pood

Hero WOD #127 – DG
10 minute AMRAP
8 TTB
35 pound Dumbbell thruster, 8 reps
35 pound Dumbbell walking lunge, 12 steps

Hero WOD #128 – TK
20 minute AMRAP
8 Strict Pull-ups
8 Box jumps, 36" box
12 Kettlebell swings, 2 pood

Hero WOD #129 – Justin
For Time
30-20-10 reps for time of:
Body-weight back squats
Body-weight bench presses
Strict pull-ups

Hero WOD #130 – Nukes
In 8 minutes. No rest between rounds.
Post run times and reps completed for each exercise.
1-mile run
315-lb. deadlifts, max reps
Then, 10 minutes to complete:
1-mile run
225-lb. power cleans, max reps
Then, 12 minutes to complete:
1-mile run
135-lb. overhead squats, max reps

Hero WOD #131 – Zembiec
5 RFT

11 back squats, 185 lb.
7 strict burpee pull-ups
400-meter run
During each burpee pull-up perform a strict push-up, jump to a bar that is ideally 12inches above your max standing reach, and perform a strict pull-up.

Hero WOD #132 – Alexander
5 RFT
31 back squats, 135 lb.
12 power cleans, 185 lb.

Hero WOD #133 – Bell
3 RFT
185-lb. deadlifts, 21 reps
15 pull-ups
185-lb. front squats, 9 reps

Hero WOD #134 – Kevin
3 RFT
185-lb. deadlifts, 32 reps
32 hanging hip touches, alternating arms
800-meter running farmer carry, 15-lb. dumbbells

Hero WOD #135 – Rocket
30 minute AMRAP
50-yard swim
10 push-ups
15 squats

Hero WOD #136 – Riley
For Time
If you've got a weight vest or body armor, wear it.
Run 1.5 miles

150 burpees
Run 1.5 miles

Hero WOD #137 – Feeks
For Time
2 x 100-meter shuttle sprint
2 squat clean thrusters, 65-lb. dumbbells
4 x 100-meter shuttle sprint
4 squat clean thrusters, 65-lb. dumbbells
6 x 100-meter shuttle sprint
6 squat clean thrusters, 65-lb. dumbbells
8 x 100-meter shuttle sprint
8 squat clean thrusters, 65-lb. dumbbells
10 x 100-meter shuttle sprint
10 squat clean thrusters, 65-lb. dumbbells
12 x 100-meter shuttle sprint
12 squat clean thrusters, 65-lb. dumbbells
14 x 100-meter shuttle sprint
14 squat clean thrusters, 65-lb. dumbbells
16 x 100-meter shuttle sprint
16 squat clean thrusters, 65-lb. dumbbells

Hero WOD #138 – Ned
7 RFT
11 body-weight back squats
1,000-meter row

Hero WOD #139 – Sham
7 RFT
11 body-weight deadlifts
100m Sprint

Chipper WODs

Chipper WOD #1 - Tuga
For time
30x Wall ball (20#/14#)
100x KB swing (53#/36#)
100x Push-ups
100x Sit-ups
100x Squats
30x Wall ball

Chipper WOD #2 - Robbie
For time
20x Back squat (225#)
40x Wall ball (20#)
60x Burpees
80x Double-unders
Run 1 mile

Chipper WOD #3
For time
Run 400m (carrying 30# sandbag)
30x Sit-ups
15x Overhead squats (95#)
25x Deadlifts (225#)
30x Pull-ups
60x Push-ups
100x Squats

Chipper WOD #4
1 round
30x Pull-ups, kipping
Run 400m
12x Pull-ups, strict
Run 800m
5x Pull-ups, weighted (40#/25#)

Run 1200m

Chipper WOD #5
For time
25x Walking lunge steps
20x Pull-ups
50x Box jumps (20 inch)
20x Double-unders
25x Ring dips
20x Knees to elbows
30x Kettlebell swings (72#)
30x Sit-ups
20x Hang squat cleans (2x35# DBs)
25x Back extensions
30x Wall ball shots (20#)
3x Rope climb ascents

Chipper WOD #6
1 round
3x Muscle-ups
5x Handstand push-ups
10x Pull-ups
20x Box jumps
30x Back extensions
40x Knees to elbows
50x Burpees
3x Muscle-ups

Chipper WOD #7 - Grand Pappy
For time
Work up to Clean & jerk 1RM
Rest 2 minutes
Run 1 mile
Rest 2 minutes

100x KB clean & jerk (44#)
Rest 2 minutes
Run 1 mile
Rest 2 minutes
100x Push-ups
Rest 2 minutes
Run 1 mile
Rest 2 minutes
100x Sit-ups

Chipper WOD #8
For time
8x Front squat (185#)
15x Burpees
7x Front squat
20x Pull-ups
6x Front squat
25x Wall-ball (20#)
5x Front squat
30x Ring dips

Chipper WOD #9
For time
Row 1000m
20x Clean & jerk (155#/105#)
30x Ring push-ups
Run 400m
30x KB swings (53#/36#)
20x Burpees
10x Pistols

Chipper WOD #10
1 round
15x Spiderman push-ups

10x Squats
15x Mountain climbers
10x Squats
15x Spartan push-ups
10x Squats
15x Hindu push-ups
10x Squats
15x Dips

Chipper WOD #11
For time
100x Squats
90x Double unders
80x Push-ups
70x Sit-ups
60x Jumping pull-ups
50x KB swings (53#/36#)
40x GHD back extensions
30x Box jumps (24/20 inch)
20x Deadlifts (225#/135#)
10x Burpees

Chipper WOD #12 - Simon Says
For time
Run 100m
25x Pull-ups
25x Push-ups
50x Deadlift (135#)
50x Box jumps (20 inch)
25x Pull-ups
25x Push-ups
Run 100m
50x Sit-ups

Chipper WOD #13
For time
Run 400m
50x Pull-ups
Run 400m
50x Push-ups
Run 400m
50x Sit-ups
Run 400m
50x Squats

Chipper WOD #14
For time
Run 1 mile
100x "Bodyblasters" (burpee + pull-up + knees to elbows)
Run 1 mile

Chipper WOD #15 - Scooter
For time
Swings are performed RKC hard style
35x KB swing (72#)
25x KB swing (88#)
15x KB swing (106#)
10x Sumo deadlift high pull (135#)
5x Deadlift (315#)
35x KB swing (72#)

Chipper WOD #16
For time
30x Back squat (245#/185#)
100m Sled drag (as heavy as possible)
50x Back extensions
20x Muscle-ups
50x Sit-ups

Run 1200m
50x Push-ups
30x Back squats

Chipper WOD #17

For time
5x Deadlift (2x bw)
10x Pull-ups
20x Burpees
30x KB swings (53#/36#)
40x Sit-ups
50x Jumping jacks
60x Squats
Row 70 calories
Run 400m

Chipper WOD #18

For max reps
6 minute cap
20x Strict pull-ups
30x Kipping pull-ups
Max reps Chest to bar pullups (reps=score)
Rest 5 minutes
6 minute cap
20x Weighted dips (90#)
30x Weighted dips (45#)
Max reps bodyweight dips (reps=score)
Rest 5 minutes
6 minute cap
20x Burpees
30x Box jumps (20 inch)
Max reps back squat @ bw (reps=score)

Chipper WOD #19 - The Big Four-two

For time
Row 42 calories
42x Push-ups
42x Sumo deadlift high-pull (95#)
42x Push press (115#)
42x Deadlifts (225#)
42x Push press
42x Sumo deadlift high-pull
42x Push-ups
Row 42 calories

Chipper WOD #20 - 2010 Barbarian Requirements

For time, 6 minute cut-off
5x Dead hang muscle-ups
45x Dips
25x Dead hang pull-ups
55x Chest-to-floor push-ups
5x Dead hang muscle-ups

Chipper WOD #21 - Barn burner

1 round
Row 250m
21x Sumo Deadlift high pull (115#/85#)
Row 500m
21x Sledgehammer tire hits
Row 750m
21x KB swing (106#/72#, RKC hard style)
Row 1000m
21x Ball slams (30#/20#)
Row 1500m

Chipper WOD #22

For time
Row 45 calories

45x DB thrusters (35#/20#)
45x Ring dips
45x Squats
Row 45 calories

Chipper WOD #23 - Szilvasi
10x Burpees
20x Clean & jerk (100#)
30x Deadlift (135#)
40x Alternating pistol squats
50x Push-ups
60x KB swings (53#)
70x Squats
80x Sit-ups
90x Wall ball (20#)
Run 1km

Chipper WOD #24
For time
40x Push-ups
20x KB swings (53#/36#)
10x Pull-ups
Run 400m
10x Pull-ups
20x KB swings (53#/36#)
40x Push-ups

Chipper WOD #25
For time
30x Pull-ups
50x KB swings (53#/36#)
75x Sit-ups
5x Handstand push-ups
30x Squats, 25x Ring dips

30x Hang power cleans (95#/65#)
15x Knees to elbows
50x Push-ups

Chipper WOD #26
For time
10x Overhead squat (155#)
10x Box jump-overs (24 inch)
10x Thruster (135#)
10x Power clean (205#)
10x Toes-to-bar
10x Burpee muscle-ups
10x Toes-to-bar
10x Power clean
10x Thruster
10x Box jump-overs
10x Overhead squat

Chipper WOD #27 - Meritorious
For time
30x Handstand push-ups
40x Pull-ups
50x Sumo deadlift high pulls
60x Sit-ups
70x Burpees

Chipper WOD #28
For time, 50x reps each
Knees to elbows
Burpees
Thrusters (45#)
Jumping ring dips
Overhead squat (45#)
KB snatches (53#/36#)

Sumo deadlift high pulls (45#)
Jumping pull-ups
Double unders

Chipper WOD #29
For time
Wear 20# vest for all movements excluding run
Run 400m
50x Pull-ups
50x Push-ups
Run 400m
50x Sit-ups
50x Squats
Run 400m

Chipper WOD #30
For time
20x Push-ups
35x Squats
20x Plyo push-ups
35x Split squats
20x Clapping push-ups
35x Broad jumps
20x Ring push-ups
35x Lateral hops (over 12" obstacle)
20x Handstand push-ups

Chipper WOD #31 - The Chuck
For time
Run 800m
21x CTB pull-ups
15x KB swings (72#)
9x Squat cleans (135#)
Run 800m

9x Squat cleans
15x KB swings
21x CTB pull-ups
Run 800m

Chipper WOD #32
For time
44x Overhead squats (45#)
44x Box jumps
44x Sit-ups
44x Hang power clean
44x Box jumps

Chipper WOD #33
For time
Run 1 mile
10x Hang squat clean (AHAP)
20x Burpees
30x Sit-ups
40x Push-ups
50x Box jumps (24/20 inch)

Chipper WOD #34 - Conky
For time
Run 400m
30x Deadlift (225#)
Run 400m
30x Power clean (185#)
Run 400m
30x Hang clean (135#)
Run 400m
30x Sumo deadlift high pull (115#)
Run 400m

Chipper WOD #35
For time
100x Sit-ups, 90x Squats
80x KB swings (53#/36#)
70x Double-unders
60x Walking lunges
50x Wall ball (20#/14#)
40x Deadlift (185#/135#)
30x Burpees
20x Push press (95#/65#)
10x Knees to elbows

Chipper WOD #36 - Lucky
For time
KB weights are 53#/36#, scale as necessary
21x KB swings
21x Push-ups
21x KB clean & jerk
21x Pull-ups
21x KB snatch
21x Sit-ups
21x KB thruster, right arm
21x Double unders
21x KB thruster, left arm

Chipper WOD #37
For time
31x Deadlifts (225#/135#)
31x Burpees
31x KB swings (53#/36#)
31x Pull-ups
31x Push-ups
31x Wall ball (20#/14#)

Chipper WOD #38
For time
100ft BB walking lunge (135#/95)
80x MB sit-ups (15#/10#)
60x Wall ball (20#/14#)
40x Chest to bar pull-ups
20 Ring dips
Run 1K

Chipper WOD #39
For time
20x KB swing (108#)
30x Single KB thruster, left arm (44#)
20x Push-ups
30x Sit-ups
20x KB sumo deadlift high pull (108#)
30x Burpees
20x Double KB snatch (2x44#)
200m Farmer's walk (2x72#)
20x KB swing (108#)

Chipper WOD #40
For time
Row 500m
25x KB swing, right hand (53#)
25x KB swing, left
Row 500m
25x KB snatch, right hand (36#)
25x KB snatch, left
Row 500m
25x KB clean & jerk, right hand (44#)
25x KB clean & jerk, left
Row 500m
25x KB swing, two-handed (72#)

25x Goblet squats (53#)

Chipper WOD #41 - WOWWSSERS
For time
Row 1000m
5x Pull-ups
10x KB swings (72#)
15x Box jumps
20x Burpees
25x Sprinter lunges
30x Push-ups
35x KB snatch (53#)
40x Walking lunges
45x/leg Flutter kicks
40x Squats

Chipper WOD #42
1 round
Run 1200m
100x Push-ups
150x Sit-ups
200x Squats
Run 1200m

Chipper WOD #43
For time
100x Squats
100x Pull-ups
200x Push-ups
300x Squats
100x Walking lunge steps

Chipper WOD #44 - Sweet pea
1 round

50x Double unders
10x Box jumps
40x Double unders
20x Box jumps
30x Double unders
30x Box jumps
20x Double unders
40x Box jumps
10x Double unders
50x Box jumps

Chipper WOD #45 - Vern
For time
50x Pull-ups
Run 400m
100x Push-ups
Run 400m
150x Sit-ups
Run 400m
200x Squats
Run 400m
250x Double-unders

Chipper WOD #46
For time
Run 1 mile
60x Push-ups
40x Ring dips
20x Handstand push-ups
10x/leg Pistols
20x Handstand push-ups
40x Ring dips
60x Push-ups
Run 1 mile

Chipper WOD #47
For time
20x Power clean (115#/75#)
10x Handstand push-ups
20x Hang power clean
30x KB swings (53#/36#)
20x Power clean
30x Burpees
20x Hang power clean
10x Strict pull-ups
20x Power clean

Chipper WOD #48
For time
50x Sit-ups
50x Double unders
50x Sit-ups
50x Walking lunge steps
50x Sit-ups, 50x Burpees
50x Sit-ups

Chipper WOD #49
For time
5x DB thrusters (55#/30#)
10x Squat jumps
20x Weighted walking lunge steps (55#/30# DBs)
30x Mountain climbers
40x Paralette push-ups with feet on 16 inch box
50x Pull-ups
60x Sit-ups

Chipper WOD #50
For time

50x Double KB front squat (36#/24#)
Row 1000m
100x Double-unders
Run 1600m
50x KB swings (53#/36#)

Chipper WOD #51
For time
Run 800m
30x Overhead squats (45#)
30x Box jumps
30x Squats
30x Broad jumps
Run 800m

Chipper WOD #52
For time
10x Muscle-ups
30x KB swings (53#/36#)
Row 40 calories
60x Push press(65#/45#)
20x Push-ups
40x KB swings
Run 400m
100x Jumping jacks
30x Sit-ups
15x Pull-ups
50x Double unders
10x Deadlifts (225#/155#)

Chipper WOD #53 - **Frogman's** Christmas
For time
100x Dead hang pull-ups
250x Push-ups

500x Sit-ups
Run 3 miles

Chipper WOD #54
For time
50x Squats
25x Push-ups
50x Pistols
25x Fingertip push-ups
50x Jumping alternating lunges
25x knuckle push-ups
50x Walking lunges
25x Diamond push-ups

Chipper WOD #55 - Louis Hell
For time
Run 400m between each exercise
20x Jump squats
20x KB swings (53#)
20x Burpees
20x Overhead squat (95#)
20x Muscle-ups
20x Box jump (24 inch)
20x each leg KB overhead walking lunges (36#)

Create Your Own WODs

Sometimes you may need or want to create your own WOD. Two things that you want to remember, no matter the approach you take to your workouts, is that the workouts should be short in duration and challenging in intensity. There are three main categories that you can choose from when selecting what exercises you will use on a particular day: gymnastics (i.e, bodyweight drills or calisthenics), metabolic conditioning (i.e. CV), and weightlifting (i.e. exercises with barbells, kettlebells, medicine balls, and dumbbells). You may choose to do a workout by selecting an exercise from either one, two or three categories.

You can keep your workout simple by selecting a single exercise from one of these three categories. Should you choose an exercise from the gymnastics category, this is a good opportunity to work on your technique. If you prefer a metabolic conditioning workout, you can lower the resistance (intensity), but increase the duration. A single element weightlifting workout would also be adequate for enhancing your strength.

As you've seen the 1,000 examples in this book, there are countless ways to make a WOD. Each can be tailored to suit your needs.

A WOD that includes two exercises should include exercises from two different categories (i.e. weightlifting and cardio, or weightlifting and gymnastics). This type of workout is typically completed for time, with an established goal for the number of repetitions or sets that should be completed. The intensity for this type of workout should be moderate to challenging. Also, try to minimize recovery time between.

You may also choose to create a WOD with elements from all three categories. Typically, you will want to designate a time limit and complete as many rounds as possible of the three exercises. Predetermine the number of repetitions for each exercise. This type of workout should be at least moderately challenging.

No matter what you choose to do for your WOD on a given day, make sure to allow yourself adequate time to warm-up and cool-down. Make sure that your workouts vary from day to day. And always keep track of your workouts so that you can track your progress as you get stronger.

I've given you 1,000 workouts that you can try yourself or use as inspiration to create your own. Get inspired, have fun and be creative with your WOD choices!

Cool Down

The cool-down portion of a workout is an often neglected but very important part of any Cross Training workout. At the very least you should walk around and sip water. You do not want to sit or lay down right after your training session. It is bad for your body both physiologically and psychologically.

Psychologically, you are Cross Training to become empowered and stronger. If you sprawl out on the floor and sit with your head hanging, those are signs of defeat. You kicked that workout's butt! Hold your head high in your success.

Physiologically, it can be very bad for your body to just stop after a workout. Remember that these are incredibly intense workouts that increase your heart rate and the volume of blood travelling through your body to your heart. As you are working out, your body is overcoming gravity to bring blood flow from your extremities to your heart so that your vital organs and tissue receive enough blood to support the high intensity level of the workout. When you just stop after your workout, your heart rate does not have time to come down properly. However, at the same time, you are no longer generating enough power to bring that blood from your extremities to the heart. This can lead to fainting or dizziness because blood is pooling in your extremities. Also, not properly cooling down can lead to a buildup of lactic acid in your system, causing not only faster fatigue, but also a potential decrease in your athletic performance.

So just remember the importance of your cool down. Stay on your feet; walk around; do an easy jog if you want to; stretch. Make sure that you allow your heart rate to slow down and your muscles to recover. In addition to the short term improvements in recovery, you will also see a long term increase in athletic performance.

Summary

Whether you were a beginner or a seasoned Cross Training athlete when you purchased this book, by now you have most likely challenged your body and mind in ways you never knew you could, and have achieved a higher level of fitness and confidence than you ever imagined possible.

As you continue on your Cross Training journey, I would urge you to try new things. If there is a subcategory that you did not try before because it is not your favorite, go ahead and give it a try anyway. You may surprise yourself as to what you will enjoy. This book can remain your reference as you expand your fitness practice, no matter at what level you may find yourself.

Remember to always warm-up, cool down and listen to your body; but never stop challenging yourself. Cross Training is high intensity, but it is nothing that you cannot handle! And do not forget to keep a record of how far you come as you complete your WODs. There is nothing more satisfying than looking back and realizing that you have just killed a PR (personal record) when you have completed a challenging workout. Continue to live in health and have fun!

Finally, if you enjoyed this book, then please be kind enough to leave a review for it on Amazon so that we can share the benefits of Cross Training with even more people. It'd be greatly appreciated.

Thank you and keep killing those PRs!

TJ Williams

About the Author

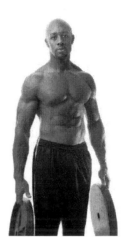

"Discipline is the bridge between goals and accomplishment"
~Jim Rohn

We all possess the potential to achieve great things in life. Big goals are common place in today's society, but only a small percentage of people will take the action required to attain such feats.

TJ Williams is a gym owner and one of the top Personal Trainers in North America. He's worked with hundreds of clients to meet their physical needs in aesthetics, functional fitness and high level performance.

TJ was born and raised in Daytona Beach, Florida. He spent most of his childhood playing sports and keeping fit. He went on to study Exercise Science at Florida State University and became a Personal Trainer. He now owns multiple gyms in the east coast of America, writes fitness books and dedicates his time to transforming people's physiques and lives.

When he's not training or writing, TJ enjoys spending time with his friends and family, playing Soduko, and travelling.

Another Title by TJ Williams

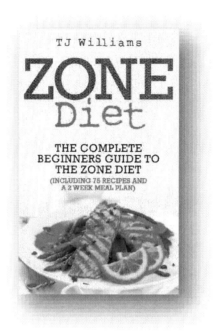

Zone Diet: The Complete Beginners Guide to the Zone Diet

(Including 75 recipes and a 2 week meal plan)

While you might have heard people talk about the 'Paleo Diet', which is a very popular nutrition strategy, you might not be as familiar with another useful dietary routine by the name of the 'Zone Diet'. This is a diet form that primarily consists of consuming foods with high protein and low carbohydrates on 5 equally balanced meals that span throughout the day.

This book will introduce you to the Zone Diet, its benefits, and how to implement it into your life with 75 recipes and a 2 week meal plan.

Made in the USA
Columbia, SC
18 January 2024